T0263464

Men's Health

Guest Editor

STEVEN A. KAPLAN, MD

UROLOGIC CLINICS OF NORTH AMERICA

www.urologic.theclinics.com

February 2012 • Volume 39 • Number 1

SAUNDERS an imprint of ELSEVIER, Inc.

W.B. SAUNDERS COMPANY
A Division of Elsevier Inc.

1600 John F. Kennedy Blvd. • Suite 1800 • Philadelphia, PA 19103-2899

http://www.theclinics.com

UROLOGIC CLINICS OF NORTH AMERICA Volume 39, Number 1
February 2012 ISSN 0094-0143, ISBN-13: 978-1-4557-3948-6

Editor: Stephanie Donley
Developmental Editor: Donald Mumford

© **2012 Elsevier Inc. All rights reserved.**

This journal and the individual contributions contained in it are protected under copyright by Elsevier, and the following terms and conditions apply to their use:

Photocopying
Single photocopies of single articles may be made for personal use as allowed by national copyright laws. Permission of the Publisher and payment of a fee is required for all other photocopying, including multiple or systematic copying, copying for advertising or promotional purposes, resale, and all forms of document delivery. Special rates are available for educational institutions that wish to make photocopies for non-profit educational classroom use. For information on how to seek permission visit www.elsevier.com/permissions or call: (+44) 1865 843830 (UK)/(+1) 215 239 3804 (USA).

Derivative Works
Subscribers may reproduce tables of contents or prepare lists of articles including abstracts for internal circulation within their institutions. Permission of the Publisher is required for resale or distribution outside the institution. Permission of the Publisher is required for all other derivative works, including compilations and translations (please consult www.elsevier.com/permissions).

Electronic Storage or Usage
Permission of the Publisher is required to store or use electronically any material contained in this journal, including any article or part of an article (please consult www.elsevier.com/permissions). Except as outlined above, no part of this publication may be reproduced, stored in a retrieval system or transmitted in any form or by any means, electronic, mechanical, photocopying, recording or otherwise, without prior written permission of the Publisher.

Notice
No responsibility is assumed by the Publisher for any injury and/or damage to persons or property as a matter of products liability, negligence or otherwise, or from any use or operation of any methods, products, instructions or ideas contained in the material herein. Because of rapid advances in the medical sciences, in particular, independent verification of diagnoses and drug dosages should be made.

Although all advertising material is expected to conform to ethical (medical) standards, inclusion in this publication does not constitute a guarantee or endorsement of the quality or value of such product or of the claims made of it by its manufacturer.

Urologic Clinics of North America (ISSN 0094-0143) is published quarterly by Elsevier Inc., 360 Park Avenue South, New York, NY 10010-1710. Months of issue are February, May, August, and November. Business and Editorial Offices: 1600 John F. Kennedy Blvd., Suite 1800, Philadelphia, PA 19103-2899. Periodicals postage paid at New York, NY and additional mailing offices. Subscription prices are $339.00 per year (US individuals), $561.00 per year (US institutions), $396.00 per year (Canadian individuals), $687.00 per year (Canadian institutions), $492.00 per year (foreign individuals), and $687.00 per year (foreign institutions). Foreign air speed delivery is included in all *Clinics* subscription prices. All prices are subject to change without notice. **POSTMASTER:** Send address changes to *Urologic Clinics of North America*, Elsevier Health Sciences Division, Subscription Customer Service, 3251 Riverport Lane, Maryland Heights, MO 63043. Customer Service: 1-800-654-2452 (US). From outside the United States, call 1-314-447-8871. Fax: 1-314-447-8029. E-mail: JournalsCustomerServiceusa@elsevier.com (for print support) and JournalsOnlineSupport-usa@elsevier.com (for online support).

Reprints. For copies of 100 or more, of articles in this publication, please contact the Commercial Reprints Department, Elsevier Inc., 360 Park Avenue South, New York, New York 10010-1710. Tel.: 212-633-3813; Fax: 212-462-1935; E-mail: reprints@elsevier.com.

Urologic Clinics of North America is covered in MEDLINE/PubMed (*Index Medicus*), *Excerpta Medica, Current Contents/Clinical Medicine, Science Citation Index,* and *ISI/BIOMED.*

Printed and bound by CPI Group (UK) Ltd, Croydon, CR0 4YY
Transferred to Digital Print 2012

Contributors

GUEST EDITOR

STEVEN A. KAPLAN, MD
E. Darracott Vaughan Jr Professor of Urology,
Director, Iris Cantor Men's Health Center;
Chief, Institute for Bladder and Prostate Health,
Weill Cornell Medical College, Cornell
University, New York, New York

AUTHORS

BILAL CHUGHTAI, MD
Fellow, James Buchanan Brady Foundation,
Department of Urology, Weill Medical College
of Cornell University, New York, New York

CHRISTOPHER M. DEIBERT, MD, MPH
Department of Urology, Herbert Irving Cancer
Center, New York, New York

**S. LARRY GOLDENBERG, CM, OBC, MD,
FRCSC**
Professor and Head, Department of Urologic
Sciences, University of British Columbia,
Vancouver, British Columbia, Canada

BRIAN T. HELFAND, MD, PhD
Fellow, Department of Urology, Northwestern
University Feinberg School of Medicine,
Chicago, Illinois

TERRY W. HENSLE, MD, FACS, FAAP
Department of Urology, Hackensack University
Medical Center, Hackensack, New Jersey

DEBORAH A. JOHNSON, BA
Executive Director, Washington State Urology
Society, Mill Creek, Washington; Board
Member, Northwest Chapter, Association for
Strategic Planning, Los Angeles, California

STEVEN A. KAPLAN, MD
E. Darracott Vaughan Jr Professor of Urology,
Director, Iris Cantor Men's Health Center;
Chief, Institute for Bladder and Prostate Health,
Weill Cornell Medical College, Cornell
University, New York, New York

RICHARD K. LEE, MD, MBA
Assistant Professor, James Buchanan Brady
Foundation, Department of Urology,
Weill Medical College of Cornell University,
New York, New York

KEVIN R. LOUGHLIN, MD, MBA
Professor of Surgery (Urology), Harvard
Medical School, Brigham and Women's
Hospital, Boston, Massachusetts

DANIEL J. MAZUR, MD
Resident, Department of Urology,
Northwestern University Feinberg School
of Medicine, Chicago, Illinois

KEVIN T. MCVARY, MD, FACS
Professor, Department of Urology,
Northwestern University Feinberg School
of Medicine, Chicago, Illinois

MARTIN M. MINER, MD
Associate Professor of Family Medicine and
Urology, Department of Family Medicine;
Co-Director, The Men's Health Center, The
Miriam Hospital, The Warren Alpert School
of Medicine, Brown University, Providence,
Rhode Island

MARK A. MOYAD, MD, MPH
Jenkins/Pokempner Director of Preventive &
Alternative Medicine, Department of Urology,
University of Michigan Medical Center, Ann
Arbor, Michigan; Consulting Director of
Medical Education & Research, Eisenhower
Wellness Institute, Eisenhower Medical Center,
Rancho Mirage, California

RICHARD S. PELMAN, MD
Clinical Professor of Urology, Department of
Urology, University of Washington School of
Medicine, Seattle, Washington; Chair,
Committee on Men's Health, Washington State
Urology Society, Washington; Chair, State
Society Network, American Association of
Clinical Urologists

JACOB RAJFER, MD
Professor of Urology, Department of Urology,
David Geffen School of Medicine at University
of California, Los Angeles, California; Chief of

Urology, Division of Urology, Harbor-UCLA
Medical Center, Torrance, California

JEREMY B. SHELTON, MD
Department of Urology, David Geffen School
of Medicine at University of California,
Los Angeles, California

ALEXIS E. TE, MD
Professor of Urology, James Buchanan Brady
Foundation, Department of Urology,
Weill Medical College of Cornell University,
New York, New York

Contents

An office evaluation of men's health in primary care requires a thorough understanding of the implications of male sexual dysfunctions, hypogonadism, and cardiometabolic risk stratification and aggressive risk management. The paradigm of the men's health office visit in primary care is the recognition and assessment of male sexual dysfunction, specifically erectile dysfunction, and its value as a signal of overall cardiometabolic health, including the emerging evidence linking low testosterone and the metabolic syndrome. Indeed, erectile dysfunction may now be thought of as a harbinger of cardiovascular clinical events and other systemic vascular diseases in some men.

Many men do not take recommended measures to screen for prostate cancer. Additionally, insurance companies have not always reimbursed for cancer screenings. This article highlights the Washington State Urology Society's efforts at improving patient outcomes through legislatively mandated cancer screenings.

Since the first "test tube" baby, Louise Brown, was born on July 25, 1978, there have been unbridled advances in the diagnosis and treatment of male infertility. There have now been more than 4 million individuals born using assisted reproductive technologies, with approximately 170,000 coming from donated oocytes and embryos. There have been many other significant achievements in the treatment of male infertility in recent decades, which are included in this review.

The Men's Health Initiative of British Columbia (MHIBC) was created as a large-scale umbrella initiative aimed at connecting the dots by identifying, coordinating, and consolidating the existing foci of excellence across the many domains of male health in the province, enabling widespread community and professional education, risk assessment, prevention-promotion, screening, and early diagnosis. The MHIBC will reach out to men across all ages, races, and socioeconomic groups and will apply a male lens to current and future health research, health promotion, awareness, and health policy development.

The metabolic syndrome (MetS) has become one of the major public health challenges worldwide. Emerging data have now clearly demonstrated its impact on male sexual function. The MetS appears to be strongly related to erectile dysfunction as well as hypogonadism. Few randomized studies exist to guide treatment of sexual dysfunction related to MetS; rather, most studies have been observational in nature. Medical therapy has formed the mainstay of treatment, with the advent of surgical intervention as a more recent phenomenon.

Androgen deficiency in aging men is common, and the potential sequelae are numerous. In addition to low libido, erectile dysfunction, decreased bone density, depressed mood, and decline in cognition, studies suggest strong correlations between low testosterone, obesity, and the metabolic syndrome. Because causation and its directionality remain uncertain, the functional and cardiovascular risks associated with androgen deficiency have led to intense investigation of testosterone replacement therapy in older men. Although promising, evidence for definitive benefit or detriment is not conclusive, and treatment of late-onset hypogonadism is complicated.

As men age, there is an increase in the frequency of pathologic diseases affecting the genitourinary tract. Most notable among these changes are the rising prevalence of lower urinary tract symptoms (LUTS) secondary to benign prostatic hyperplasia (BPH) and erectile dysfunction (ED). The pathogenesis of these conditions seems to be multifactorial and includes age-related changes in the nervous system and neuroregulatory factors, such as nitric oxide and RhoA/Rho-kinase. Various pharmacologic agents that target these pathways, such as α-blockers and PDE-5is, underscore the contribution of neuroregulatory factors on the development of LUTS/BPH and ED.

The primary cause of mortality in most developed countries is cardiovascular disease, which is the primary cause of death in the largest clinical studies of male health conditions. There are simplistic correlations between heart health and male-specific diseases. Clinicians need to motivate and provide a simplistic and realistic set of lifestyle, dietary supplement, and prescription drug recommendations to men to affect all-cause morbidity and mortality. This article provides recommendations to assist the clinician and patient to make practical changes that may be accomplished in a short period of time, and should provide tangible overall benefit for men's health.

Congenital abnormalities of the genitourinary system have a definable durable impact on the adult lives of those individuals affected, despite prompt and appropriate surgical and medical intervention during infancy and childhood. Three abnormalities are described, including relatively common problems of the newborn male, such as hypospadias and cryptorchidism, as well as a less common issue, posterior urethral valves. An understanding and awareness of the consequences of these 3 congenital abnormalities is paramount for the long-term care of the pediatric patient as he transitions to adolescence and adulthood.

GOAL STATEMENT

The goal of *Urologic Clinics of North America* is to keep practicing urologists and urology residents up to date with current clinical practice in urology by providing timely articles reviewing the state of the art in patient care.

ACCREDITATION

The *Urologic Clinics of North America* is planned and implemented in accordance with the Essential Areas and Policies of the Accreditation Council for Continuing Medical Education (ACCME) through the joint sponsorship of the University of Virginia School of Medicine and Elsevier. The University of Virginia School of Medicine is accredited by the ACCME to provide continuing medical education for physicians.

The University of Virginia School of Medicine designates this enduring material activity for a maximum of 15 *AMA PRA Category 1 Credit*(s)™ for each issue, 60 credits per year. Physicians should claim only the credit commensurate with the extent of their participation in the activity.

The American Medical Association has determined that physicians not licensed in the US who participate in this CME enduring material activity are eligible for a maximum of 15 *AMA PRA Category 1 Credit*(s)™ for each issue, 60 credits per year.

Credit can be earned by reading the text material, taking the CME examination online at http://www.theclinics.com/home/cme, and completing the evaluation. After taking the test, you will be required to review any and all incorrect answers. Following completion of the test and evaluation, your credit will be awarded and you may print your certificate.

FACULTY DISCLOSURE/CONFLICT OF INTEREST

The University of Virginia School of Medicine, as an ACCME accredited provider, endorses and strives to comply with the Accreditation Council for Continuing Medical Education (ACCME) Standards of Commercial Support, Commonwealth of Virginia statutes, University of Virginia policies and procedures, and associated federal and private regulations and guidelines on the need for disclosure and monitoring of proprietary and financial interests that may affect the scientific integrity and balance of content delivered in continuing medical education activities under our auspices.

The University of Virginia School of Medicine requires that all CME activities accredited through this institution be developed independently and be scientifically rigorous, balanced and objective in the presentation/discussion of its content, theories and practices.

All authors/editors participating in an accredited CME activity are expected to disclose to the readers relevant financial relationships with commercial entities occurring within the past 12 months (such as grants or research support, employee, consultant, stock holder, member of speakers bureau, etc.). The University of Virginia School of Medicine will employ appropriate mechanisms to resolve potential conflicts of interest to maintain the standards of fair and balanced education to the reader. Questions about specific strategies can be directed to the Office of Continuing Medical Education, University of Virginia School of Medicine, Charlottesville, Virginia.

The faculty and staff of the University of Virginia Office of Continuing Medical Education have no financial affiliations to disclose.

The authors/editors listed below have identified no professional or financial affiliations for themselves or their spouse/partner:
Bilal Chughtai, MD; Christopher M. Deibert, MD, MPH; Stephanie Donley, (Acquisitions Editor); Brian T. Helfand, MD, PhD; Terry W. Hensle, MD; Deborah A. Johnson, BA; Steven A. Kaplan, MD (Guest Editor); Richard K. Lee, MD, MBA; Daniel J. Mazur, MD; and Jeremy B. Shelton, MD.

The authors/editors listed below identified the following professional or financial affiliations for themselves or their spouse/partner:
S. Larry Goldenberg, CM, OBC, MD, FRCSC is on the Advisory Board for GSK Canada and Sanofi Aventis Canada.
Kevin R. Loughlin, MD, MBA is a consultant for Certus Biomedical, Taris, and Tengion, and is a Board Member of Predictive Biosciences.
Kevin T. McVary, MD is a consultant for Lilly/ICOS, Watson, Neotract, NIDDK, Allergan, and GSK; is on the Speakers' Bureau for GSK; and is an industry funded research/investigator for Allergan, Johnson & Johnson, and Lilly/ICOS.
Martin M. Miner, MD is a consultant for Abbott, Auxillium, and BI, and receives research support from GSK.
Mark A. Moyad, MD, MPH is a consultant for Abbott Labs, Embria Health Sciences, Farr Labs, Guthy Renker, and NBTY; is on the Speakers' Bureau for Abbott Labs; and receives royalties from Guthy Renker.
Richard S. Pelman, MD owns stock in Pfizer, Inc, is a consultant for Astellas, Abbott, and Light Sciences Corp., and is on the Speakers' Bureau for Astellas and GSK.
Jacob Rajfer, MD receives research funding from Allergan and POM Wonderful.
William Steers, MD (Test Author) is employed by the American Urologic Association, is a reviewer and consultant for NIH, and is an investigator for Allergan.
Alexis E. Te, MD is an industry funded research/investigator for NIH, Allergan, Pfizer, Inc., and Neotract, and is a consultant and is on the Speakers' Bureau for American Medical Systems.

Disclosure of Discussion of Non-FDA Approved Uses for Pharmaceutical Products and/or Medical Devices
The University of Virginia School of Medicine, as an ACCME provider, requires that all faculty presenters identify and disclose any off-label uses for pharmaceutical and medical device products. The University of Virginia School of Medicine recommends that each physician fully review all the available data on new products or procedures prior to clinical use.

TO ENROLL

To enroll in the Urologic Clinics of North America Continuing Medical Education program, call customer service at 1-800-654-2452 or visit us online at www.theclinics.com/home/cme. The CME program is available to subscribers for an additional fee of $207.00.

Urologic Clinics of North America

THE CLINICS ARE NOW AVAILABLE ONLINE!

Access your subscription at:
www.theclinics.com

Preface
Men's Health

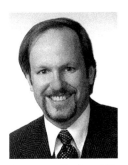

Steven A. Kaplan, MD
Guest Editor

The evolving nature of gender health is an emerging and fertile area for urologists. In an era of diminished resources, there is great opportunity for urologists to broaden their scope and how they interact with both their peers and their patients. Given the ominous increase in both obesity and diabetes in the United States and the increasingly recognized association between metabolic dysfunction and urologic health, there is a great opportunity for urologists to acquaint themselves better with multiple health issues from cradle to grave. For example, lower urinary tract symptoms (LUTS) and sexual dysfunction are highly prevalent in men; these associations between LUTS and sexual dysfunction are independent of age and comorbidities, such as heart disease and diabetes. Evidence linking disorders of the prostate and bladder with LUTS and sexual dysfunction is irrefutable, but the contribution of metabolic, cardiovascular, and endocrine factors cannot be discounted. What is the underlying association? Moreover, in an era where the prevalence of metabolic syndrome is increasing particularly in the face of an epidemic of obesity, where do urologists fit in?

This issue of *Urologic Clinics* is dedicated to exploring how we can better hone both our diagnostic and our therapeutic skills in various disorders of adolescent and aging males. Moreover, how we interact with primary care physicians to enhance the care of men will be of great benefit to our specialty. Urologists and their leadership organizations are dedicated to the promotion of and awareness of both long-term health and disease prevention and to the education of men regarding preventive intervention, healthy lifestyles, and the benefits of entering the health care system in a timely manner. Ultimately, urologists want to be both advocates and facilitators for men's health. This includes recognizing Urology as an important specialty and the need for our specialty to adapt to changing patients, medical practice, and health care environments. I congratulate all the authors for their superb contributions and hope this issue will be of great interest and information to our readers.

Steven A. Kaplan, MD
Department of Urology
Weill Cornell Medical College
New York Presbyterian Hospital
F9 - West, 525 East 68th Street
New York, NY 10065, USA

E-mail address:
kaplans@med.cornell.edu

Urol Clin N Am 39 (2012) xi
doi:10.1016/j.ucl.2011.10.001
0094-0143/12/$ – see front matter © 2012 Elsevier Inc. All rights reserved.

Men's Health in Primary Care: An Emerging Paradigm of Sexual Function and Cardiometabolic Risk

Martin M. Miner, MD

KEYWORDS

- Primary care • Men's health • Erectile dysfunction
- Endothelial cell dysfunction

WHY MEN'S HEALTH?

Gender-based medicine, specifically recognizing the differences in the health of men and women, drew much attention in the 1990s. The National Institutes of Health's Office of Research on Women's Health was established in 1990, and in 1994 the Food and Drug Administration (FDA) created an Office of Women's Health, resulting in a dramatic increase in the quantity and quality of research devoted to examining numerous aspects of women's health such that today women's health research is clearly mainstream.[1]

While decades of research have yielded many important findings about health and disease in men, this knowledge has not resulted in the benefits expected. Men are still less likely than women to seek medical care, and are nearly half as likely as women to pursue preventive health visits or undergo screening tests.[2] Recent data indicate that 68.6% of men aged 20 years and older are overweight,[3] and life expectancy of men continues to trail that of women, by 5.3 years in 2003.[4]

Men's Health as a concept and discipline is in a historic state compared with women's health. Most clinicians and the public consider Men's Health to be a field concerned only with the prostate and sexual function. Men's health has recently become a hot topic in these specific areas with large amounts of dollars being spent on remedies for prostate health, improved urinary flow, and enhanced erections, with a smaller amount directed to overall improved health.[5]

Men do not use or react to health services in the same way as women.[6] Men are less likely to go to health care providers for preventive health care visits.[7] Men are also less likely to follow medical regimens, and are less likely to achieve control with long-term therapeutic treatments.[8,9] The Commonwealth Fund did a mass survey and found that "an alarming proportion of American men have only limited contact with physicians and the health care system generally. Many men fail to get routine check-ups, preventive care, or health counseling and they often ignore symptoms or delay seeking medical attention when sick or in pain."[10] This report concludes by noting the need for increased efforts to address the special needs of men as well as attitudes toward health care. Men are more likely to be motivated to visit the doctor for diseases that specifically affect men most, such as baldness, sports injuries, or erectile dysfunction (ED). The presentation of a man to the clinician's office with a sexual health complaint can present an opportunity for a more complete evaluation, most notably with the complaint of ED. In a landmark article published in December, 2005, Thompson and colleagues[11] confirmed what had been long believed: that ED is a sentinel marker and risk factor for future cardiovascular

Department of Family Medicine and Urology, The Men's Health Center, The Miriam Hospital, 164 Summit Avenue, The Warren Alpert School of Medicine, Brown University, Providence, RI 02906, USA
E-mail address: Martin_Miner@Brown.edu

Urol Clin N Am 39 (2012) 1–23
doi:10.1016/j.ucl.2011.09.003
0094-0143/12/$ – see front matter © 2012 Elsevier Inc. All rights reserved.

events. After adjustment, incident ED occurring in the 4300 men without ED at study entry enrolled in the Prostate Cancer Prevention Trial (PCPT) was associated with a hazard ratio of 1.25 for subsequent cardiovascular events during the 9-year study follow-up (1994–2003). For men with either incident or prevalent ED, the hazard ratio was 1.45. Thus, men with ED are at risk for developing cardiac events over the next 10 years, with ED as strong a risk factor as current smoking or premature family history of cardiac disease. Never before has the association of ED or a male sexual dysfunction been so strongly linked as a harbinger of cardiovascular clinical events in men.

WHO IS THE MEN'S HEALTH DOCTOR: PRIMARY CARE PHYSICIAN VERSUS PRIMARY CARE PHYSICIAN MEN'S HEALTH SUBSPECIALIST VERSUS UROLOGIST

While urologists are typically thought of as *men's doctors* as obstetricians/gynecologists are considered *women's doctors*, the issue remains as to who is to shoulder this responsibility in the decades to come, regardless of reform. Will it be a shared care approach, including clear communication between urologists and primary care clinicians, and vice versa, or do we need to enhance this relationship or specialty? Do we need to create separate "Centers of Excellence" for men's health, as the author has strived to do at the Miriam Hospital and Warren Alpert School of Medicine of Brown University? Do we need to establish Men's Health Fellowships for nonurologists dealing more with the issues of "medical urology?" Having practiced as a primary care clinician for over 25 years before opening this Center of Men's Health 2 years ago (composed of urological, psychological, and comprehensive cardiometabolic medical evaluation), I (the author of this article) feel a need to reflect on past and present experience.

First, what I miss most from routine primary care is longitudinal care compressed into a series of vignettes, no greater than 10 to 15 minutes, spanning the course of decades. There is a sense of familiarity and rapport that is immediate and refreshed in each visit. The patient's concerns are varied, often multiple and unpredictable, and require rapid thinking, concise summations, and treatment plans. I came to treasure these encounters, and felt validated and loved by my patients.

Second, I have struggled to morph myself into a subspecialist from a primary care clinician. In my former life, I dictated or charted solely for myself and my cross-covering peers, and not for review as a referring subspecialist. With this additional role, my language must be supportive, direct, and nonprovocative. I must recognize the boundaries of my work, make recommendations, but recognize that as one primary care provider/subspecialist speaking to another, the tone and content of my charting has to focus almost entirely on evidence-based medicine, noting the studies rationalizing my suggesting the use of an angiotensin receptor blocker/angiotensin-converting enzyme for this patient's hypertension and sexual function, or the addition of bupropion to a selective serotonin reuptake inhibitor for antidepressant-induced sexual dysfunction. I must take caution to recommend a slow taper of the noncardioselective β-blocker in the post–myocardial infarction patient, now 3 years out, and replacement with perhaps a more sexually friendly and endothelial enhancing drug such as nebivolol. When I suggest a means to improve diabetic control, including focus on lifestyle and diet, or perhaps a more aggressive stance to managing dyslipidemia, I must proceed with caution. Who am I and what training do I have to make these recommendations? Most internists to whom I correspond do not know of the years spent at American Urological Association (AUA) meetings, boards, committees, and self-developed preceptorships I have encountered. Nor do they know of the tumultuous path to election to the Sexual Medicine Society of North America's fellowship and Board of Directors, and membership to the AUA's Committee on Men's Health. To them, I can easily be accused of assuming primary care for the patient. And indeed, there may be some accuracy to this claim in the post–radical prostatectomy "penile-rehab" patient when I am aggressively suggesting control of cardiometabolic risk factors and neuromodulation with statins, to name examples. It is clear that without the background knowledge, the primary care clinician may misinterpret my goals and rationale.

Therefore, not to be accused of "co-opting" primary care patients from one clinician to another, I must presently recognize when it is time to step aside, relinquish my duties and contact with patients with whom I have become quite fond of over the past 2 years during their rehabilitation, and steadfastly refuse overtures to become their primary care physician. My appeal may be that I am focusing on a single, highly personal medical problem, their sexual dysfunction, and not the usual laundry-list of the standard primary care visit: type 2 diabetes; hypertension; dyslipidemia; sprinkled with a bit of generalized anxiety.

Our interactions in the Men's Health Center are not replicated in the world of volume primary care, and I am the first to acknowledge the wondrous reality of my situation and its accompanying depth of interaction and emotional content. Indeed, my focus is often as much "lifestyle coach" as it is cardiometabolic medicine.

Which system is better? This is yet to be known. In my former life as primary care physician whereby I incorporated this interest of sexual medicine into my daily practice, I saw on average 34 to 36 patients per day, short-changing much thought and discussion to remain respectful of patients' (and my) time, yet bringing sessions to a close with a warm touch of the arm or shoulder, and some genuine laughter. Contrast this to the Men's Health Center, where each patient has a similar "template" and complaints are relatively a known quantity, as are patients' stories. Though I approach the second with passion, excitement, and "reflective listening," maintaining eye contact, we may not know the answer to this question until we have objective outcomes. However, intuitively I feel that this combination of urologist-andrologist/internal medicine-family physician/psychologist-sex therapist is most unusual and offers a unique opportunity to enhance gender-specific care. Routinely individuals see two providers at the initial visit: urologist/internist or internist/psychologist. I am kidded by the urologists; my notes still begin with a story: married, divorced, or living with wife and children; partnered or semi-partnered; open-married or close-married; job satisfaction; life stresses; and partner relationship. Again, the good in this model is my focus on the "whole" male.

Historically, the office visit for a man complaining of sexual dysfunction focused solely on ED, and this was the narrow definition of men's health. Over the past several years epidemiologic studies and novel data have mandated that the primary care clinician redirect this office visit to include a broader definition of both sexual function and dysfunction: premature ejaculation, libido and hypogonadism, and the potential medical causes of each of these. Given the value of Thompson's study, a cardiovascular assessment and an even broader cardiometabolic risk assessment should be performed in light of the data suggesting that ED may be a sentinel sign of cardiovascular disease (CVD).

The next section provides the rationale for this global assessment paradigm in primary care and other men's health topics including sexual issues, but does not include other pertinent topics of men's health including affective and mood disorders, domestic and partner violence, and other gender-specific issues. Disparities among multicultural differences in men's health, as it exists in a socioeconomic means and disease prevalence among various multiethnic groups, are beyond the scope of this article.

THE PRIMARY CARE OFFICE VISIT AS A PORTAL TO MEN'S HEALTH: MALE SEXUAL EVALUATION
Erectile Dysfunction

Definition
For years, the terms impotence and ED had been used interchangeably to denote the inability of a man to achieve or maintain erection sufficient to permit satisfactory sexual intercourse.[12] Social scientists objected to the impotence label, because of its pejorative implications and lack of precision.[13] A National Institutes of Health (NIH) Consensus Development Conference[14] advocated that ED be used in place of the term impotence. ED or impotence was now defined as "the inability of the male to achieve an erect penis as part of the overall multifaceted process of male sexual function." This definition deemphasizes intercourse as the sine qua non of sexual life, and gives equal importance to other aspects of male sexual behavior.

Epidemiology
It is estimated that at least 10 to 20 million American males suffer from ED.[15,16] Laumann and colleagues[16] have shown that the prevalence of male sexual dysfunction approaches 31% in a population survey of approximately 1400 men aged 18 to 59 years; in the National Health and Social Life Survey hypogonadism (5%), ED (5%), and premature ejaculation (21%) were the 3 most common male sexual dysfunctions noted.

The Massachusetts Male Aging Study,[15] a large epidemiologic study, asked men between the ages of 40 and 70 years to categorize their erectile function as either completely, moderately, minimally, or not impotent. Fifty-two percent of the sample reported some degree of ED. This study demonstrated that ED is an age dependent disorder; "between the ages of 40–70 years the probability of complete impotence tripled from 5.1% to 15%, moderate impotence doubled from 17 to 34% while the probability of minimal impotence remained constant at 17%." By age 70, only 32% portrayed themselves as free of ED. Finally, cigarette smoking increased the probability of total ED in men with treated heart disease, hypertension, or untreated arthritis. It similarly increased the probability for men on cardiac, antihypertensive, or vasodilator medications.

After the data were adjusted for age, men treated for diabetes (28%), heart disease (39%), and hypertension (15%) had significantly higher probabilities for ED than the sample as a whole (9.6%). Men with untreated ulcer (18%), arthritis (15%), and allergy (12%) were also significantly more likely to develop ED. Although ED was not associated with total serum cholesterol, the probability of dysfunction varied inversely with high-density lipoprotein (HDL) cholesterol.[16]

Certain classes of medication were related to increased probability for total ED. The percentage of men with complete dysfunction taking hypoglycemic agents (26%), antihypertensives (14%), vasodilators (36%), and cardiac drugs (28%) was significantly higher than the sample as a whole (9.6%).[16]

More recent data added greater depth to the United States national estimates of ED. The National Health and Nutrition Examination Survey (NHANES), conducted by the National Center for Health Statistics, collected data by household interview supplemented by medical examination. The sample size for the entire survey for the 2-year period was 11,039, with a response rate of 71.1% for men 20 years and older. Data include medical histories in which specific queries are made regarding sexual function. In men 20 years and older, ED affected almost 1 in 5 respondents. Hispanic men were more likely to report ED (odds ratio [OR], 1.89), after controlling for other factors. The prevalence of ED increased dramatically with advanced age; 77.5% of men 75 years and older were affected. In addition, there were several modifiable risk factors that were independently associated with ED, including diabetes mellitus (OR, 2.69), obesity (OR, 1.60), current smoking (OR, 1.74), and hypertension (OR, 1.56).[17]

Relationship between ED and cardiovascular disease

Data specific to ED and related diseases has emerged, and serves to support the relationship between ED and CVD. Seftel and colleagues[18] quantified the prevalence of diagnosed hypertension, hyperlipidemia, diabetes mellitus, and depression in male health plan members (United States) with ED, using a nationally representative managed care claims database that covered 51 health plans with 28 million lives for 1995 through 2002. Crude population prevalence rates in this study population were 41.6% for hypertension, 42.4% for hyperlipidemia, 20.2% for diabetes mellitus, 11.1% for depression, 23.9% for hypertension and hyperlipidemia, 12.8% for hypertension and diabetes mellitus, and 11.5% for hyperlipidemia and depression.[18] The crude age-specific prevalence rates varied across age groups significantly for hypertension (4.5%–68.4%), hyperlipidemia (3.9%–52.3%), and diabetes mellitus

(2.8%–28.7%), and significantly less for depression (5.8%–15.0%). Region-adjusted population prevalence rates were 41.2% for hypertension, 41.8% for hyperlipidemia, 19.7% for diabetes mellitus, and 11.9% for depression. Of 87,163 patients with ED (32%) had no comorbid diagnosis of hypertension, hyperlipidemia, diabetes mellitus, or depression. These data suggested and confirmed that hypertension, hyperlipidemia, diabetes mellitus, and depression were prevalent in patients with ED.[18] This evidence supported the proposition that ED shares common risk factors with these 4 concurrent conditions, supporting the view that ED could be viewed as a potential observable marker for these concurrent CVD risk conditions.

Further epidemiologic data have suggested that ED may be an early marker for actual CVD. Min and colleagues[19] studied 221 men referred for stress myocardial perfusion single-photon emission computed tomography (MPS) commonly used to diagnose and stratify CVD. It was found that 55% of the patients had ED, and that these men exhibited more severe coronary heart disease (MPS summed stress score >8) (43% vs 17%; $P<.001$) and left ventricular dysfunction (left ventricular ejection fraction <50%) (24% vs 11%; $P = .01$) than those without ED. These data suggested that ED might be an independent predictor of more severe coronary artery disease and high-risk MPS findings.

Evolving data support the ED-cardiovascular paradigm. A sample of nearly 4000 Canadian men,[20] aged 40 to 88 years, seen by primary care clinicians reported ED with the use of the International Index of Erectile Function (IIEF). The presence of CVD or diabetes mellitus increased the probability of ED, and among those individuals without CVD or diabetes mellitus the calculated 10-year Framingham coronary risk increase and fasting glucose level increase were independently associated with ED. ED was also independently associated with undiagnosed hyperglycemia (OR, 1.46), impaired fasting glucose (OR, 1.26) and the metabolic syndrome (OR, 1.45).

The prospective analysis discussed in the introduction by Thompson and colleagues[11] of the nearly 9500 men randomly assigned to the placebo arm of the PCPT revealed that men with ED are at significantly greater risk ($P<.001$) of having a cardiovascular event—angina, myocardial infarction, or stroke—than those without ED. Furthermore, the findings indicate that the relationship between incident ED (the first report of ED of any grade) and CVD is comparable with that associated with current smoking, family history of myocardial infarction, or hyperlipidemia.

Subsequent to the Thompson analysis and lending further support to the idea of ED as a precursor of CVD, Montorsi and colleagues[21] in the COBRA study investigated 285 patients with coronary artery disease (CAD). A key finding is that nearly all patients who developed CAD symptoms experienced ED symptoms first, on average 2 to 3 years beforehand. Finally, ED and CVD share a similar pathogenic involvement of the nitric oxide pathway, leading to impairment of endothelium-dependent vasodilatation (early phase) and structural vascular abnormalities (late phase).[22] Thus, ED may be considered as the clinical manifestation of a vascular disease affecting the penile circulation; likewise, angina pectoris is the clinical manifestation of a vascular disorder affecting coronary circulation.

Moreover, while there is growing opinion that ED is an index of subclinical coronary disease and a precursor of cardiovascular events, a variety of mechanisms have been proposed.[21,23] ED could be a predictor because it leads to depression, which leads in turn to increased cardiac risk. Or men with ED may have higher body mass index (BMI) or other comorbidities that leads to both ED and CAD.[16,24]

As the Thompson study[11] lent further support to the notion that ED is predominantly a disease of vascular origin, with endothelial cell dysfunction as the unifying link, investigations in diabetics have also supported this concept, and in fact suggest that ED is a predictor of future cardiovascular events in this group. Gazzaruso and colleagues[25] recruited 291 type 2 diabetic men with silent CAD and found that those who developed major adverse cardiac events over the course of approximately 4 years were more likely to have ED (61.2%) than those who did not (36.4%). Through further multivariate analysis, ED remained an important predictor of adverse cardiac events, and although diabetics have a high risk of CVD, the risk is even higher in those who develop ED.

Ma and colleagues[26] studied 2306 diabetic men with no clinical evidence of CAD, of whom 27% had ED. Over the course of approximately 4 years, the incidence of coronary heart disease was greater in men with ED (19.7/1000 person-years) than in men without ED (9.5/1000 person-years). After adjustments for other covariates, including age, duration of disease, antihypertensive agents, and albuminuria, ED remained an independent predictor of coronary heart disease (hazard ratio [HR] 1.58, 95% confidence interval [CI] 1.08–2.30, $P = .018$).

Therefore, because ED and silent CAD are prevalent in the diabetic population, this should move all health care providers in primary care to inquire about sexual function in the diabetic patient, and aggressively treat cardiovascular risk factors including dyslipidemia and hypertension. Indeed, the Second Princeton Consensus Panel[24] on sexual activity and cardiac risk published recommendations for the individual with established CAD or suspected CAD related to estimated risk for cardiovascular events, and in those individuals of intermediate or indeterminate risk (no overt cardiac symptoms and 3 or more cardiovascular risk factors including sedentary lifestyle; moderate stable angina; recent myocardial infarction <6 weeks; New York Heart Association Class II heart failure; prior stroke, transient ischemic attack (TIA) or history of peripheral vascular disease) should receive further cardiac evaluation to delineate the presence and severity of coronary disease.

It is therefore recommended that physicians screen the ED patient for vascular disease, and because ED often coexists with the comorbidities of diabetes (3–4-fold incidence), hypertension, or dyslipidemia, screening in the primary care clinician's office for ED should occur with the management of each of these comorbiities.[27]

What does ED tell us in the nondiabetic population?

What about the nondiabetic, noncomorbid population? What does the presence of ED suggest in the lower-risk male population not yet studied to date? To this point, Inman and colleagues[28] biennially screened a random sample of more than 1400 community-dwelling men who had regular sexual partners and no known CAD for the presence of ED over a 10-year period. Men were followed from the fourth screening round (1996) of the Olmsted County Urinary Symptoms and Health Status among Men Study until the first occurrence of an incident cardiac event or the last study visit (December 31, 2005). Men with prevalent ED at study onset were excluded from the analyses. Multivariate proportional hazard regression models were used to assess the association of the covariates of age, diabetes, hypertension, smoking status, and BMI with ED. Unlike the Thompson study or others already noted, the participants of this study were not a highly selected subset of the general male population and older than 55 years, but more representative of a normal (albeit predominantly Caucasian) group of men. In addition, erectile function of the study participants was assessed by an externally validated questionnaire, the Brief Male Sexual Function Inventory (BMSFI),[29] a self-reported questionnaire comprising 11 items rated on a scale of 0 to 4, with higher scores representing better sexual function.

During the 10-year follow-up period, ED was modeled as a time-dependent covariate that allowed each patient's ED status to change over time, with results stratified by 10-year age periods and adjusted for diabetes, hypertension, smoking status, and BMI.

Baseline prevalence of ED was 2% for 40-year-olds, 6% for 50-year-olds, 17% for 60-year-olds, and 39% for men older than 70. New ED developed in 6.4% at 2 years with increases of approximately 5% in each subsequent 2-year interval over the 10-year period of follow-up. Incident ED was more common in patients with higher cardiovascular risk and older age.[28]

Overall, new incident CAD developed in 11% of men over the 10-year follow-up period, with approximately 15% due to myocardial infarction, 79% to angiographic anomalies, and 6% to sudden death. The cumulative incidence of CAD was strongly influenced by patient age. CAD incidence densities per 1000 person-years for men without ED were 0.94 (age 40–49), 5.09 (age 50–59), 10.72 (age 60–69), and 23.30 (age 70+). For men with ED, the incidence densities for CAD were 48.52 (age 40–49), 27.15 (age 50–59), 23.97 (age 60–69), and 29.63 (age 70+) (**Fig. 1**).[28]

Is ED a greater predictor of cardiovascular disease in the younger (age <60 years) male?

The meaning of these findings is most significant. While ED and CAD may be different manifestations of an underlying vascular pathology, when ED occurs in a younger man (age <60) it is associated with a marked increase in the risk of future cardiac events whereas in older men it appears to have less prognostic value. The importance of this study cannot be understated. Whereas ED had little relationship with the development of incident cardiac events in men aged 70 years and older, it was associated with a nearly 50-fold increase in the 10-year incidence in men 49 years and younger. This finding raises the possibility of a "window of curability" whereby progression of cardiac disease might be slowed or halted by medical intervention. Younger men with ED could provide the ideal populations for future studies of primary cardiovascular risk prevention.[30]

Why younger than older men? Clearly there is a higher incidence of psychogenic ED in younger men, and the argument can be made that all ED has a psychological component. However, in the younger male with more than one cardiovascular risk factor, his ED and CAD may be different manifestations of an underlying vascular pathology. ED appears to precede symptoms of CAD in patients with a vascular etiology. Montorsi and colleagues[31] suggest that this phenomenon relates to the caliber of the blood vessels. For example, the penile artery has a diameter of 1 to 2 mm, whereas the proximal left anterior descending coronary artery is 3 to 4 mm in diameter. An equally sized atherosclerotic plaque burden in the smaller penile arteries would more likely compromise flow earlier and cause ED compared with the same amount of plaque in the larger coronary artery causing angina. In another plausible explanation, Inman and colleagues[28] suggest greater impairment in arterial endothelial cell function with age. The repetitive pulsations to which the large central arteries are subjected over their lifespan lead to fatigue and fracture of the elastic lamellae, resulting in increased stiffness.[32] Ultimately small arteries such as the pudendal and penile arteries begin to degenerate and end-organ ischemia results. In the younger male with ED, impaired vasodilation of a penile artery is more likely to lead to ED, even in the absence of atherosclerotic plaque narrowing the lumen, than in the same scenario in the coronary arteries leading to symptoms of angina.[31]

Hacket[27] goes further to elaborate that the treatment of ED with phosphodiesterase type 5 inhibitors as a class, and particularly in studies demonstrated with sildenafil and tadalafil, has been shown to dilate epicardial coronary arteries, improve endothelial dysfunction, and inhibit platelet activation in patients with CAD.[33,34] The availability of effective, noninvasive treatment methods, which have a significant impact on the quality of life of men with ED, means that an

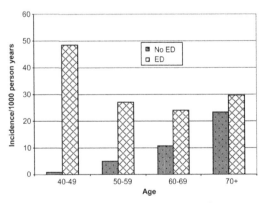

Fig. 1. Incidence per 1000 person-years of ED associated with coronary artery disease densities (incidence densities in patients with and without ED). (*Data from* Inman BA, Sauver JL, Jacobson DJ, et al. A population-based longitudinal study of erectile dysfunction and future coronary artery disease. Mayo Clin Proc 2009;84(2):108–13; with permission.)

increase in the diagnosis of ED could benefit a large number of men and their partners, and potentially improve the pathology leading to the condition itself.

Although ED is associated with cardiovascular risk factors and atherosclerosis, it is not known whether the presence of ED is predictive of future events in individuals with known CVD. Bohm and colleagues[34] evaluated whether ED is predictive of mortality and cardiovascular outcomes, and because inhibition of the renin-angiotensin system in high-risk patients reduces cardiovascular events, wished to establish whether there are protective effects of the pharmacologic inhibition of this system. Therefore, the investigators additionally tested the effects on ED of randomized treatments with telmisartan, ramipril, and the combination of the two drugs (ONTARGET), as well as with telmisartan or placebo in patients who were intolerant of angiotensin-converting enzyme inhibitors (TRANSCEND).

In a prespecified substudy, 1549 patients, of whom 842 had a history of ED at baseline and were slightly older (65.8 years vs 63.6 years, $P<.0001$) with a higher prevalence of hypertension, stroke/TIA, diabetes mellitus, and lower urinary tract symptoms (LUTS), underwent double-blind randomization, with 400 participants assigned to receive ramipril, 395 telmisartan, and 381 the combination thereof (ONTARGET), as well as 171 participants assigned to receive telmisartan and 202 placebo (TRANSCEND).[34] ED was evaluated at baseline, at 2-year follow-up, and at the penultimate visit before closeout. Because of the nature of the study population, incident ED or new-onset ED clearly was small. However, either baseline or incident ED was predictive of all-cause death (HR 1.84, 95% CI 1.21–2.81, $P = .005$) and the composite primary outcome (HR 1.42, 95% CI 1.04–1.94, $P = .029$), which consisted of cardiovascular death (HR 1.93, 95% CI 1.13–3.29, $P = .016$), myocardial infarction (HR 2.02, 95% CI 1.13–3.58, $P = .017$), hospitalization for heart failure (HR 1.2, 95% CI 0.64–2.26, $P = .563$), and stroke (HR 1.1, 95% CI 0.64–1.9, $P = .742$). The study medications did not influence the course or development of ED.

ED is a potent predictor of all-cause death and the composite of cardiovascular death, myocardial infarction, stroke, and heart failure in men with CVD. Trial treatment with either telmisartan or ramipril did not significantly improve or worsen ED.[34] This finding is somewhat surprising given these agents' beneficial effects on endothelial cell function.

Whether ED is only a risk marker or may even be considered a "CAD risk equivalent" (an independent risk factor) is not yet fully clarified; yet there is evidence to consider all men with ED younger than 60 years to be at risk of CVD until proved otherwise.[35,36] However, given the high prevalence of ED in the middle-aged population, a systematic cardiologic screening would not be cost effective. Therefore, it is crucial to identify ED patients at high risk for occult CAD or acute coronary events, or both. The task for the clinician is to identify those patients with ED who may be at intermediate or high risk for subsequent CVD.[35,36] A reasonable first step is to estimate, through one of several risk assessment office-based approaches, the subject's own relative and absolute risk of a cardiovascular event (usually in the following 10 years). Lloyd-Jones and colleagues[37] recommend incorporating a stepwise approach to cardiovascular risk stratification, with the Framingham criteria used for all patients and the lifetime analysis added for those predicted to be at low 10-year risk. This type of systematic analysis and use of the Princeton II guidelines[38] can help the practitioner distinguish between the presence of organic and cardiovascular risk versus largely psychological etiology in this middle-aged ED patient.

The aforementioned studies suggest that a presentation of ED should trigger an assessment of cardiovascular risk factors and, if appropriate, vigorous intervention.

Psychosocial morbidity of ED

The impact of ED frequently extends beyond a man's physical function; it can have a psychological effect on a man and his partner, producing disquiet. Consequently, the emotional toll that ED can have on men and their partners should be considered in the diagnosis and management of ED. A global survey of 13,618 men from 29 countries found that 13% to 28% have ED,[39] and a survey of 1481 men in the Netherlands[40] found that, of those with ED, 67% were bothered by it and 85% wanted help for their condition. Left untreated, the emotional distress associated with ED can significantly affect important psychosocial factors, including self-esteem and confidence, and damage personal relationships.[41,42] In their Consensus Development Panel on Impotence, the NIH recommended that studies continue to investigate the social and the psychological effects of ED in patients and their partners.[14] However, there are few data on the effect of ED and its treatment on trouble associated with ED, which may be due in part to the absence of data from an instrument designed to assess the bother or distress that is specific to ED.

Summary and recommendations

ED is a common men's sexual health complaint, increases in prevalence with aging, is bothersome, and is a future marker for CVD. A verbal inquiry or a brief written 5-item survey (SHIM)[43] can be used to quantify the degree of ED, and thereby the concomitant risk of CVD. ED is associated with hypertension, diabetes, depression, hyperlipidemia, smoking,[43,44] sedentary lifestyle,[45] and obesity. Thus, the man presenting to the clinician complaining of ED should have these areas explored. In addition to defining and characterizing the specific sexual complaint (discussed later), a brief cardiovascular assessment of risk factors, including smoking, lifestyle and exercise, diet, blood pressure, lipids, weight, and distress, should all be part of the initial evaluation. A World Health Organization consensus panel has deliberated and agreed that these recommendations about associating ED with the need for a CVD evaluation are reasonable.[46]

Hypogonadism (Testosterone Deficiency)

Definition

The US FDA has accepted a total testosterone (TT) level of 300 ng/dL as the lower limit of normal for serum testosterone levels. Others have challenged this level, citing a variety of reasons as to why a level of 300 ng/dL is not a true reflection of hypogonadism. Reasons include a lack of age-specific norms, a lack of evidence that 300 ng/dL is a proper number, and a lack of symptoms reflecting what the testosterone level represents. Clinicians have gravitated to the term "late-onset hypogonadism" to suggest that an older group of men might be a more appropriate group of individuals on whom we should focus with respect to testosterone deficiency. An international consensus statement[47] (published in 3 to 4 journals simultaneously) has offered the following guidance.

1. Definition of late-onset hypogonadism (LOH): A clinical *and* biochemical syndrome associated with advancing age and characterized by typical symptoms and a deficiency in serum testosterone levels. It may result in significant detriment in the quality of life and adversely affect the function of multiple organ systems.
2. LOH is a syndrome characterized primarily by:
   a. The easily recognized features of diminished sexual desire (libido) and erectile quality and frequency, particularly nocturnal erections
   b. Changes in mood with concomitant decreases in intellectual activity, cognitive functions, spatial orientation ability, fatigue, depressed mood, and irritability

   c. Sleep disturbances
   d. Decrease in lean body mass with associated diminution in muscle volume and strength
   e. Increase in visceral fat
   f. Decrease in body hair and skin alterations
   g. Decreased bone mineral density resulting in osteopenia, osteoporosis, and increased risk of bone fractures.

Epidemiology

A recent review of this topic sheds light on the epidemiology of hypogonadism.[48] In healthy, young eugonadal men, serum testosterone levels range from 300 to 1050 ng/dL, but decline with advancing age, particularly after 50 years.[49–53] Using a serum testosterone level of 325 ng/dL, the Baltimore Longitudinal Study of Aging (BLSA) reported that approximately 12%, 20%, 30%, and 50% of men in their 50s, 60s, 70s, and 80s, respectively, are hypogonadal.[50]

The Hypogonadism in Males (HIM) study[52] estimated the prevalence of hypogonadism (TT <300 ng/dL) in men aged 45 years or older visiting primary care practices in the United States. A blood sample was obtained between 8 AM and noon and was assayed for TT, free testosterone (FT), and bioavailable testosterone (BAT). Common symptoms of hypogonadism, comorbid conditions, demographics, and reason for visit were recorded. Of 2162 patients, 836 were hypogonadal, with 80 receiving testosterone. The crude prevalence rate of hypogonadism was 38.7%. Similar trends were observed for FT and BAT.[52]

Longitudinal and cross-sectional studies have demonstrated annual testosterone decrements of 0.5% to 2% with advancing age.[51–55] The rate of decline in serum testosterone in men appears to be largely dependent on their age at study entry. In the BLSA,[50] the average decline was 3.2 ng/dL per year among men aged 53 years at entry. On the other hand, the New Mexico Aging Process Study of men 66 to 80 years old at entry showed a decrease in serum testosterone of 110 ng/dL every 10 years.[53] Although serum testosterone levels are generally measured in the morning when at peak, this circadian rhythm is often abolished in elderly men.[55]

Testing for hypogonadism and determining who requires testosterone replacement

The recommendations of the International Society of Andrology, International Society for the Study of the Aging Male, and European Association of Urology[47] note that in patients at risk for or suspected of hypogonadism in general and LOH in particular, a thorough physical and biochemical workup is mandatory and in particular, the following biochemical investigations should be done:

1. A serum sample for total T determination and sex hormone–binding globulin (SHBG) should be obtained between 07.00 and 11.00 hours. The most widely accepted parameters to establish the presence of hypogonadism are the measurement of TT and FT calculated from measured TT and SHBG or measured by a reliable FT dialysis method.
2. There are no generally accepted lower limits of normal, and it is unclear whether geographically different thresholds depend on ethnic differences or on the physician's perception. There is, however, general agreement that TT levels above 12 nmol/L (346 ng/dL) or FT levels above 250 pmol/L (72 pg/mL) do not require substitution. Similarly, based on the data from younger men, there is consensus that serum TT levels below 8 nmol/L (231 ng/dL) or FT below 180 pmol/L (52 pg/mL) require substitution. Since symptoms of testosterone deficiency become manifest between 12 and 8 nmol/L, trials of treatment can be considered in those in whom alternative causes of these symptoms have been excluded. (Since there are variations in the reagents and normal ranges among laboratories, the cutoff values given for serum T and FT may have to be adjusted depending on the reference values given by each laboratory.)
3. If testosterone levels are below or at the lower limit of the accepted normal adult male values, it is recommended to perform a second determination together with assessment of serum luteinizing hormone and prolactin.
4. A clear indication, based on a clinical picture together with biochemical evidence of low serum testosterone, should exist prior to the initiation of testosterone substitution.

The Endocrine Society has recently published its set of guidelines, entitled "Testosterone Therapy in Adult Men with Androgen Deficiency Syndromes: An Endocrine Society Clinical Practice Guideline,"[56] which has been updated this year.[57]

The Endocrine Society recommends making a diagnosis of androgen deficiency only in men with consistent symptoms and signs and unequivocally low serum testosterone levels. These recommendations include the measurement of morning TT level by a reliable assay as the initial diagnostic test. Confirmation of the diagnosis is suggested, by repeating the measurement of morning TT and in some patients by measurement of FT or BAT level, using accurate assays. Overall the Society recommends testosterone therapy for symptomatic men with androgen deficiency, who have low testosterone levels, to induce and maintain secondary sex characteristics and to improve their sexual function, sense of well-being, muscle mass and strength, and bone mineral density.

These recommendations prohibit starting testosterone therapy in patients with breast or prostate cancer, a palpable prostate nodule, or induration or prostate-specific antigen (PSA) greater than 3 ng/mL without further urological evaluation, erythrocytosis (hematocrit >50%), hyperviscosity, untreated obstructive sleep apnea, severe LUTS with International Prostate Symptom Score (IPSS) greater than 19, or class III or IV heart failure. When testosterone therapy is instituted, they suggest aiming at achieving testosterone levels during treatment in the mid-normal range with any of the approved formulations, chosen on the basis of the patient's preference, consideration of pharmacokinetics, treatment burden, and cost. Men receiving testosterone therapy should be monitored using a standardized plan.

In 2004, the Institute of Medicine (IOM) reviewed the current state of knowledge about testosterone therapy in older men, concluding:

As the FDA-approved treatment for male hypogonadism, testosterone therapy has been found to be effective in ameliorating several symptoms in markedly hypogonadal males. Researchers have carefully explored the benefits of testosterone therapy particularly placebo-controlled randomized trials, in the population of middle aged or older men who do not meet all the clinical diagnostic criteria for hypogonadism but who may have testosterone levels in the low range for young adult males and show one or more symptoms that are common to both aging and hypogonadism.[58]

The IOM further concluded that "assessments of risks and benefits have been limited and uncertainties remain about the value of this therapy in older men."[58]

Shames and colleagues[59] of the US FDA conclude that:

We support the right of individual physicians to treat patients based on their own knowledge or advice from known experts in the field. However, patients should be able to choose therapies based on accurate and evidence-based medical information and consultation with well-informed health care providers. Clinical guidelines and patient guides should be based on solid clinical evidence and must convey this information clearly and accurately to physicians and patients.[59]

The IOM report also cited evidence for a possible association of low endogenous testosterone with components of the metabolic syndrome,[58] which has been defined in various ways but generally includes insulin resistance, obesity, abnormal lipid profiles, and borderline or overt hypertension.[58] Recent studies have confirmed that hypogonadism predisposes men to insulin resistance, obesity, abnormal lipid profiles, and borderline or overt hypertension.[58] In 2005, a systematic review concluded that evidence linking hypogonadism and metabolic syndrome is of sufficient strength that the definition of the metabolic syndrome in men may be expanded in the future to include hypogonadism as a diagnostic parameter.[60]

Among men with diabetes, the prevalence of hypogonadism has been reported to range from 20% to 64%.[61,62] A systematic review and meta-analysis of 43 prospective and cross-sectional studies concluded that men with type 2 diabetes had significantly lower concentrations of testosterone than did men with normal fasting glucose.[63]

Recent clinical studies have confirmed that TT is inversely associated with BMI, waist-hip ratio, and percentage body fat and insulin resistance.[64–67] Insulin resistance among hypogonadal men may be an indirect effect of changes in body composition, inhibition of lipoprotein lipase, or decreased circulating free fatty acids.[68,69] A series of data analyses from the Kuopio Ischemic Heart Disease Risk Factor Study, conducted in Finland, reported that nondiabetic men were nearly fourfold more likely to develop metabolic syndrome if they were hypogonadal,[70] twice as likely to develop diabetes or metabolic syndrome within an 11-year period if they were in the lowest quartile for testosterone levels,[71] and up to 2.9 times as likely to develop hypogonadism during the 11-year follow-up period if they had metabolic syndrome at baseline.[72] Therefore, it is highly evident that low testosterone is positively correlated with the onset of metabolic syndrome, and perhaps of type 2 diabetes. This correlation may have clinical and economic significance because of the high prevalence and substantial costs of diabetes and metabolic syndrome in the United States.[73–75]

Potential reversibility of the link between metabolic syndrome and hypogonadism was suggested by an observational study and a recent interventional study. In the observa-

tional study, new-onset hypogonadism was 5.7 to 7.4 times more common among men with metabolic syndrome at baseline and at final visit, and approximately 3 times more common among men who also had new-onset metabolic syndrome; however, no increased risk of hypogonadism was observed among men who had metabolic syndrome at baseline that had resolved by the final visit.[76] In the interventional study of 58 obese men with metabolic syndrome, the prevalence of hypogonadism (TT <317 ng/dL) was 48% at baseline, 9% after the men lost an average of 16.3 kg on a very low-calorie diet, and 21% when men regained approximately 2 kg on average during a 12-month weight maintenance program.[77] Significant improvements in insulin sensitivity, fasting glucose, HDL levels, and triglycerides were observed at the end of each treatment phase.[78]

Emerging evidence suggests that the opposite is true as well—namely, that testosterone replacement therapy may ameliorate some of the elements of metabolic syndrome—but results of these studies have been mixed (Table 1). Several studies have reported that testosterone replacement therapy in hypogonadal men decreased body weight, waist-hip ratio, and body fat, and improved glycemic control, insulin resistance, and/or the lipid profile.[77–82] However, some of these studies reported that one or more of the parameters of metabolic syndrome were not significantly improved by testosterone replacement therapy. Additional long-term studies are needed to elucidate the role of testosterone replacement therapy in improving body composition and clinical outcomes associated with the metabolic syndrome.

Summary and recommendations

It seems reasonable that irrespective of the testosterone level that is chosen by the clinician for the diagnosis of hypogonadism, certain hypogonadism-associated symptoms should be sought out and detailed in the patient record. For those clinicians unfamiliar with these symptoms, the questionnaires (Table 2) should suffice. Caution must be the guide here as we make slow, steady progress in understanding testosterone replacement issues. Prostate gland monitoring and PSA can be followed safely by the recommendations in Box 1. The overall recommendations noted in the two sets of guidelines already outlined provide helpful guidance.

Table 1
Testosterone and the reversibility of metabolic syndrome: studies published since the 2003 IOM report

Authors,[Ref.] Year	Study Design	Key Findings
Fukui et al,[67] 2003	Cross-sectional study of 253 men with type 2 diabetes (mean ± SD age, 62.0 ± 9.9 y)	Correlations with total testosterone: ↓ patient age ↓ age of diabetes onset ↓ duration of type 2 diabetes ↑ total cholesterol ↓ intima media thickness ↔ cardiovascular disease ↔ cerebral infarction ↔ coronary artery disease
Corrales et al,[62] 2004	Cross-sectional study of 55 diabetic men aged >50 y, 8 aging controls, and 32 young controls	Correlations with total testosterone: ↔ fasting glucose ↔ fructosamine ↔ insulin ↔ C-peptide ↑ HbA$_{1c}$ Prevalence of hypogonadism 20%–55% among diabetic men, depending on the criteria used
Pitteloud et al,[64] 2005	Cross-sectional study of 60 men with normal glucose tolerance (n = 27), impaired glucose tolerance (n = 12), or type 2 diabetes (n = 21)	Correlations with total testosterone: ↓ insulin resistance ↓ body mass index ↓ waist-hip ratio ↓ body fat % Hypogonadal men (total testosterone <9.7 nmol/L) were twice as insulin resistant 90% of hypogonadal men met the criteria for metabolic syndrome
Kalme et al,[66] 2005	Cross-sectional study of 335 men aged 70–89 y	Correlations with total testosterone: ↓ glucose ↓ insulin ↓ age ↓ body mass index ↓ triglycerides ↑ HDL cholesterol
Basaria et al,[101] 2006	Cross-sectional study of 18 hypogonadal, androgen-deprived men with prostate cancer; 17 eugonadal men with prostate cancer; and 17 eugonadal healthy men	Correlations with total testosterone: ↓ glucose ↓ insulin ↓ insulin resistance ↓ leptin
Smith et al,[65] 2006	Single-arm treatment study of leuprolide depot and bicalutamide in 25 nondiabetic men with locally advanced or recurrent prostate cancer	Androgen blockade increased HbA$_{1c}$, insulin level, insulin resistance, total cholesterol, HDL cholesterol, and triglycerides

Abbreviations: HbA$_{1c}$, glycosylated hemoglobin; HDL, high-density lipoprotein; ↑, positive correlation; ↓, negative correlation; ↔, no correlation.

From Miner M, Seftel A. Testosterone and aging: what have we learned since the IOM report and what lies ahead. IJCP 2007;61(4):622–32; with permission.

Table 2
Questionnaires used to diagnose androgen deficiency in aging males

Androgen Deficiency in Aging Males (ADAM) Questionnaire[124,a]	Massachusetts Male Aging Study (MMAS) Questionnaire[88,b]
1. Do you have a decrease in libido (sex drive)?	Libido—"How frequently do you feel sexual desire" (1–8)
2. Do you have a lack of energy?	Erectile dysfunction—13-item composite (1–4)
3. Do you have a decrease in strength and/or endurance?	Depression—antidepressant use (yes/no)
4. Have you lost height?	Lethargy—past week (1–4)
5. Have you noticed a decreased "enjoyment of life"?	Inability to concentrate—past week (1–4)
6. Are you sad and/or grumpy?	Sleep disturbance—past week (1–4)
7. Are your erections less strong?	Irritability—past week (1–4)
8. Have you noted a recent deterioration in your ability to play sports?	Depressed mood—past week (1–4)
9. Are you falling asleep after dinner?	
10. Has there been a recent deterioration in your work performance?	

[a] A positive ADAM questionnaire was defined as a "yes" answer to Question 1, Question 7, or any 3 other questions.
[b] A positive MMAS questionnaire was defined as 3 or more positive symptoms (1–2 for libido, "yes" for antidepressant use, and 2–4 for all other items).

Box 1
Recommendations for monitoring prostate health before and during testosterone replacement therapy

Before initiating therapy

Normal digital rectal examination (DRE)

PSA <4.0 ng/mL

Evaluate individual risk of prostate cancer

During therapy

Measure PSA

At 3–6 months

Annually or semiannually as long as treatment continues

Perform DRE

Annually or semiannually as long as treatment continues

Refer for urological evaluation and possible prostate biopsy if

Prostate is abnormal on DRE

Or

PSA >4 ng/mL

or

PSA increase >1 ng/mL after 3–4 months on testosterone treatment

Or

PSA velocity >1.5 ng/mL/y or >0.75 ng/mL/y over 2 years

or

PSA velocity >0.4 ng/mL/y over an observation period of <3 years (with PSA after 6 months on testosterone therapy used as a reference point)

Data from Refs.[64,83–87]

CARDIOMETABOLIC RISK AND ED AND TESTOSTERONE DEFICIENCY: REVERSING THE RISK

ED and Cardiovascular Disease: Is Reduction of Risk Possible?

While it has been long recognized that CVD and ED were related by alterations in healthy endothelial function and vascular perfusion, it is not surprising that ED and CVD have been linked through traditional cardiovascular risk markers including cigarette smoking, hypertension, and dyslipidemia. However, the evolving concept of ED and its relationship to novel and broader cardiovascular markers tied to male waist circumference and obesity, and its association with vascular disease in other prominent vascular beds, specifically the carotid and femoral arteries, is emerging. Investigators from the Massachusetts Male Aging Study found that ED was predictive of subsequent development of the metabolic syndrome (central obesity, insulin dysregulation, abnormal lipids, and borderline hypertension). The association was greatest with men whose initial BMI was below 25 (BMI is calculated as weight in kilograms divided by height in meters squared, ie, kg/m^2).[88]

This information provides some guidance about risk reduction opportunities. Esposito and colleagues[89] determined the effect of weight loss and increased physical activity on erectile and endothelial function in obese men. The 55 men randomly assigned to the intervention group received detailed advice about how to achieve a loss of 10% or more in their total body weight by reducing caloric intake and increasing their level of physical activity. Men in the control group (n = 55) were given usual information about healthy food choices and exercise. After 2 years, BMI decreased more in the intervention group (from a mean [SD] of 36.9 [2.5] to 31.2 [2.1]) than in the control group (from 36.4 [2.3] to 35.7 [2.5]) (P<.001), as did serum concentrations of interleukin 6 (P = .03), and C-reactive protein (P = .02). The mean (SD) level of physical activity increased more in the intervention group (from 48 [10] to 195 [36] min/wk; P<.001) than in the control group (from 51 [9] to 84 [28] min/wk; P<.001). The mean (SD) IIEF score improved in the intervention group (from 13.9 [4.0] to 17 [5]; P<.001), but remained stable in the control group (from 13.5 [4.0] to 13.6 [4.1]; P = .89). In multivariate analyses, changes in BMI (P = .02), physical activity (P = .02), and C-reactive protein (P = .03) were independently associated with changes in IIEF score. The investigators concluded that lifestyle changes were associated with improvement in sexual function in about one-third of obese men with ED at baseline (**Figs. 2–4**).

Testosterone Deficiency and CVD Risk Reduction

As shown in **Fig. 2**, the relationship between testosterone deficiency and metabolic syndrome is bidirectional, complex, and involves multiple pathophysiologic pathways.[90–92] Evidence derived from epidemiologic and clinical studies[64,83–87,93–107] with testosterone replacement therapy (TRT) in hypogonadal men, as well as androgen-deprivation therapy (ADT) in prostate cancer patients, suggest that the link between testosterone deficiency and metabolic syndrome encompasses multiple pathways including increased insulin resistance, hyperglycemia, visceral fat accumulation (characterized by increased waist circumference), altered lipid profiles (dyslipidemia), increased synthesis of inflammatory cytokines,

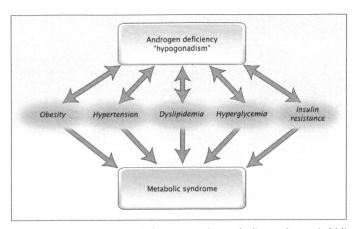

Fig. 2. The relationship between testosterone deficiency and metabolic syndrome is bidirectional. (*Data from* Traish AM, Saad F, Guay A. The dark side of testosterone deficiency: II. Type 2 diabetes and insulin resistance. J Androl 2009;30:23–32.)

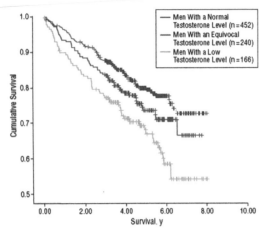

Fig. 3. Low testosterone associated with shorter survival shores. Unadjusted Kaplan-Meier survival curves for 3 T-level groups. Men with low and equivocal (one normal and one low measurement) testosterone level had a significantly shorter survival than men with normal testosterone levels (log-rank test; P = .001). Low testosterone = total testosterone <250 ng/dL (8.7 nmol/L) or free testosterone <0.75 ng/dL (0.03 nmol/L). (*Data from* Shores MM, Matsumoto AM, Sloan KL, et al. Low serum testosterone and mortality in male veterans. Arch Intern Med 2006;166:1660–5.)

and endothelial dysfunction, thus leading to vascular disease.[64,80,83–87,94,104–109]

Emerging evidence links testosterone deficiency to multiple cardiovascular risk factors including obesity, diabetes, hypertension, and altered lipid profiles, suggesting that testosterone plays an important role in the regulation of metabolic homeostasis. Testosterone deficiency has

been shown to be an independent determinant of endothelial dysfunction,[80,106,107] thus contributing to vascular pathology. TRT in hypogonadal men produced significant improvement in lipid profiles, reduced body fat percentage, increased lean muscle mass percentage, and decreased fasting glucose levels.[95,109–113]

In the Rotterdam study, a population-based prospective cohort study, relative risk of aortic atherosclerosis in men (n = 504, age ≥55 years, followed for 6.5 years) was inversely related to TT (P = .04 for trend, adjusted for covariates) and BAT (P = .004, adjusted for covariates).[93] Men in the second and third (highest) tertile of TT and BAT were protected against atherosclerotic progression compared with those in the lowest tertile (P = .02 for trend).[93]

Testosterone Deficiency and All-Cause Mortality and CVD Risk

Epidemiologic studies have identified significant associations between testosterone levels and all-cause and cardiovascular death in general populations of men 40 years or older.[114–116] Mortality rate over a mean of 4.3 years for 858 veterans with normal, equivocal (one normal, one low measurement), and low testosterone levels was 20.1%, 24.6%, and 34.9%, respectively.[114]

A larger (2314 men, age 40–79 years), longer (average 7-year follow-up) nested case-control study found that every 173 ng/dL (6 nmol/L) increase in serum testosterone was associated with a 21% lower risk of all-cause death (OR, 0.79; 95% CI 0.69–0.91, P<.01) and cardiovascular death (OR, 0.79; 95% CI 0.64–0.97, P = .02)

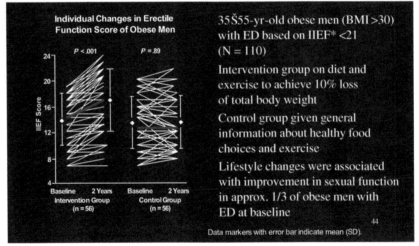

Fig. 4. Weight loss can improve sexual function in obese men. (*Adapted from* Esposito K, Giugliano F, Di Palo C, et al. Effect of lifestyle changes on erectile dysfunction in obese men: a randomized controlled trial. JAMA 2004; 291(24):2978–84; with permission.)

after excluding deaths within the first 2 years and controlling for multiple variables (age, BMI, systolic blood pressure, cholesterol, cigarette smoking, diabetes, alcohol intake, physical activity, social class, education, and SHBG).[115] Subjects had no CVD at baseline.

The Rancho Bernardo study (n = 794 men, aged 50–91 years, average follow-up 11.8 years, but up to 20 years) also found that TT and BAT were inversely related to risk of death. Men in the lowest quartile of total testosterone (<241 ng/dL [8.4 nmol/L]) were 44% more likely to die during the follow-up period compared with those in highest quartile (>370 ng/dL [12.8 nmol/L]), independent of age, BMI, waist-to-hip ratio, alcohol use, current smoking, and exercise (HR 1.44, 95% CI 1.12–1.84).[116] Additional adjustment for prevalent diabetes, CVD, or the metabolic syndrome had minimal effect on the strength of this association.[116] Low TT also predicted increased risk of death due to cardiovascular (HR 1.38, 95% CI 1.02–1.85) and respiratory disease (HR 2.29, 95% CI 1.25–4.20).[116]

Is TRT Associated with Increased Cardiovascular Events?

Chronic heart failure seems to be associated with decreased plasma testosterone levels, with approximately 25% of men with chronic heart failure found to have biochemical evidence of testosterone deficiency. Caminiti and colleagues[113] showed, in a double-blind, placebo-controlled, randomized trial of 70 elderly patients with chronic heart failure, that long-acting intramuscular testosterone supplementation on top of optimal therapy improves functional exercise capacity, muscle strength, insulin levels, and baroreflex sensitivity.[113]

In a recent trial 209 men[117] were randomly assigned to receive 10 g of transdermal gel, containing either placebo or 100 mg of testosterone, applied to the skin once daily for 6 months. This study was designed to examine the impact of testosterone repletion in men aged 65 years and older who have limitations in mobility, with end points chosen as changes in chest-press and leg-press strength and the ability to walk and climb stairs. The mean age for the men in the trial was 74 years, largely Caucasian with 56% having preexisting CVD, 85% with hypertension, and 25% diabetic. The study was terminated early because 23 of the 106 men in the testosterone group experienced adverse cardiovascular-related events including myocardial infarction, arrhythmias, and hypertension compared with 5 men of the 103 in the placebo group. At the time the study was stopped the testosterone group had significantly

greater improvements in leg-press and chest-press strength, as well as in stair climbing.

The investigators note several issues. First, the study's small size, the study's older sicker population, and the population's mobility limitations limit generalizability of the findings. It was also noted that chance could play a role in the outcomes observed, with further research needed to clarify safety issues raised by this trial.[117] Though valid, this study raises questions about the use of rather large doses of testosterone in older frail men, a group often targeted for testosterone therapy.

Can TRT Reverse or Ameliorate Metabolic Syndrome or Early Type 2 Diabetes?

The metabolic syndrome is defined as a cluster of medical conditions associated with the risk of developing insulin resistance, type 2 diabetes mellitus, and CVD, and a higher risk of incident CVD and mortality.[118] Metabolic syndrome is associated with a twofold increase of 5- to 10-year risk of CVD.[119] Furthermore, the syndrome confers a fivefold increase in risk for type 2 diabetes mellitus.[119] Despite this evidence the clinical use of this category, and in particular its utility, as a predictor of CVD has been the subject of vigorous criticism. Accordingly, recent data from the RIVANA study, a survey involving 880 community-dwelling men, supported the construct that the metabolic syndrome is not better than the sum of its components in addressing cardiovascular risk.[120]

The level of evidence supporting TRT in the treatment of metabolic syndrome, type 2 diabetes mellitus, and CVD varies because TRT administered in various formulations has differing outcomes on different aspects of clinical end points investigated. Specifically, reduction of body fat, especially intra-abdominal fat, is a key component in treating most individuals with metabolic syndrome or type 2 diabetes mellitus, as well as many patients with atherosclerotic CVD and dyslipidemia. Data linking testosterone and the metabolic syndrome raise the question of the potential impact that treating testosterone deficiency might have on the metabolic syndrome. A year-long study points to positive results. Heufelder and colleagues[112] randomized 32 hypogonadal men (total testosterone <346 ng/dL [12 nmol/L]) with newly diagnosed type 2 diabetes to diet and exercise alone or diet and exercise combined with testosterone gel therapy (50 mg once daily). All subjects met the criteria for the metabolic syndrome as defined by the National Cholesterol Education Program Adult Treatment Panel III (ATP III) as well as the more stringent International Diabetes Foundation (IDF); this definition includes stricter limits for waist circumference ($\geq$37 inches [94 cm] rather than 40 inches [101.6 cm] for European men, $\geq$31.5 inches [80 cm] rather than 35 inches [76.2 cm] for European women) and fasting plasma glucose ($\geq$100 mg/dL rather than 110 mg/dL).[121] Subjects had never received insulin or other glucose-lowering therapy, either before or during the trial,[10] and had a mean hemoglobin A_{1c} (HbA_{1c}) of 7.5.

Patients were contacted at least twice a week to encourage adherence to the exercise and diet regimen. At 52 weeks, both groups showed improvement from baseline on multiple measures including mean serum testosterone concentration, glycemic control (HbA_{1c}), insulin levels and sensitivity, and C-reactive protein levels measured by a high-sensitivity assay. The group receiving diet and exercise plus testosterone improved significantly on all aforementioned parameters in comparison with the subjects randomized to diet and exercise but without testosterone ($P<.001$ for all between-group comparisons). More than 80% of the testosterone group showed conversion of the components of the metabolic syndrome to normal values according to ATP III criteria, versus 31% of the diet and exercise alone group. At the end of the study, serum PSA concentrations were equivalent between groups, an indication of treatment safety.

Summary and Recommendations

In addition to a workup for cardiovascular risk, all men who present with ED should be assessed for the presence and severity of actual CVD and undergo hormonal testing for testosterone, if organicity is highly suspected. High-risk patients with ED should undergo exercise and/or stress testing. In this context, high-risk patients are those with ED plus diabetes, strong family history of CVD, 3 or more cardiovascular risk factors, angina, or a coronary heart disease risk equivalent.[35] Peripheral arterial disease, diabetes, and multiple risk factors with a 10-year risk of coronary heart disease greater than 20% constitute coronary heart disease risk equivaents.[99] Patients with ED and evidence of cerebrovascular disease (asymptomatic bruits and/or a history of transient ischemic events) should be assessed with carotid ultrasonography. Symptoms of circulatory insufficiency that suggest peripheral vascular disease in men with ED should be evaluated using the ankle/brachial index. Obesity, while affecting one-third of United States adults, clearly predisposes to cardiovascular risk factors including insulin resistance, hypertension, and dyslipidemia. BMI has been used as the primary standard for outcomes in studies, but alternative measures including waist circumference and waist-to-hip

ratio have demonstrated better correlations with CVD risk than BMI.[121,122] Indicators of metabolic syndrome should be identified, highlighted to patients, and treated aggressively with risk-reduction therapies, including exercise, diet, nutritional counseling, testosterone when indicated, and other pharmacotherapy.

As the author continues to note from 2006, there have been no significant randomized, placebo-controlled trials of testosterone repletion involving specific outcomes related to mortality, quality of life, fractures, fragility, cardiovascular events, or cognitive function. Much of this must be attributed to the recommendations from the IOM put forth in 2003 with the focus on smaller studies with set end points. Perhaps with the advent of these recommendations and the critical examination of the literature published in this field since 2003 and acknowledgment of the gaps in knowledge that continue to exist, this paradigm should be reexamined. It is noteworthy that these guidelines acknowledge that the strength of evidence underlying their recommendations is generally of poor quality, and editorials on this subject have also arrived at similar conclusions.[123,124] The recommendations herein are in general agreement with most published guidelines, with two primary sources of disagreement: one is that clinical presentation is emphasized over biochemical thresholds in the diagnosis of testosterone deficiency, and the second is that the author believes there is adequate evidence to support the use of TRT in selected cases for metabolic and general health indications.

SEXUAL MEDICINE HISTORY AND PHYSICAL EXAMINATION IN PRIMARY CARE

It is vital to remember that if we do not ask, men will not tell. The office evaluation consists of a series of direct questions about the nature of the sexual dysfunction complaint. Questions should be direct while inviting discussion (eg, "Do you have any concerns about your sexual functioning?") (**Box 2**). The interview should take place in a quiet room, in a nonjudgmental fashion. These men are embarrassed and often need reassurance that this topic is acceptable to discuss. The questions should be asked in a gentle manner, avoiding any gestures or posturing that might be misconstrued.

In lieu of direct questions, many clinicians prefer to provide the patient with questionnaires that delve into the specific sexual complaint.

Some examples include:

1. The Sexual Health Inventory for Men (SHIM) is a simple, 5-question instrument that inquires

Box 2
Examples of the line of inquiry into male sexual dysfunction

Characterize the sexual dysfunction

What type of sexual problem does the patient complain of?

Does he have ED?

If so, how long has he had the problem?

When was the last time he had intercourse?

When was the last time he had any sexual activity?

Does the erection problem bother him?

Does the erection problem bother his partner?

Did the problem arise suddenly (psychogenic) or has it arisen gradually?

Did the problem start when he started a new medication?

Does the problem occur with his partner only or does it also occur without his partner as well, for example with masturbation?

Does the problem occur because he has no partner or an uninterested partner?

Does he have a partner outside of his main relationship?

Can he get an erection? If so, is it firm enough for penetration?

Can he maintain the erection for intercourse?

Does he have a problem with sexual desire?

How long has he lost sexual desire?

Has he lost sexual desire with all partners?

Has he lost desire under all circumstances?

Has he lost desire because he cannot get or maintain an erection?

Has he lost desire because his partner has lost desire?

Does the patient complain of other, associated symptoms, such as being tired, loss of stamina, loss of strength, loss of muscle mass, loss of muscle tone, recent weight gain, fatigue, sleep issues?

Is the patient depressed?

Does he have a problem with ejaculation?

What type of ejaculation problem does the patient complain of?

When did the problem start?

Is the problem bothersome to the patient?

Is the problem bothersome to the partner?

Does the problem occur under all circumstances?

Box 3
Physical examination for men with sexual dysfunction

Height, weight, BMI, waist size, or waist-to-hip ratio

Blood pressure

Auscultation of heart, lungs

Check pulses

Examination of abdomen (auscultation for bruits)

Examination of penis for plaques, lesions, urethral position, elasticity, and turgor

Examination of testis for size, lumps, masses, position

Examination of rectum for sphincter tone, prostate size, masses, lesions, bulbocavernosus reflex

Brief neurologic examination

Data from Miner M, Kuritzky L. Erectile dysfunction: a sentinel marker for cardiovascular disease in primary Care. Cleve Clin J Med 2007;74:S30–7.

Box 4
Laboratory work for men complaining of ED

Fasting lipid panel

Fasting glucose

Total or free testosterone (preferably in the morning)

PSA—mandatory if considering testosterone[a] supplementation, otherwise may be optional

Optional laboratory tests:

Prolactin

Creatinine

Estradiol

Thyroid-stimulating hormone

Luteinizing hormone

25-Hydroxyvitamin D level

Urinary microalbumin

[a] There is no level 1 evidence for drawing a serum testosterone in all men with ED; a serum testosterone should be considered in men with co-morbidities associated with testosterone deficiency, or men who fail oral PDE-5 therapy.
   Data from Miner M, Kuritzky L. Erectile dysfunction: a sentinel marker for cardiovascular disease in primary Care. Cleve Clin J Med 2007;74:S30–7.

about erectile function over the previous 6 months. The SHIM is an abridged and slightly modified version of the IIEF.[43] This simpler version allows the clinician to assess male ED with great security. The SHIM is scored as follows:

Score 22–25 no ED

Score 17–21 mild ED

Score 12–16 mild to moderate

Score 8–11 moderate

Score 0–7 severe ED (in my experience consider psychogenic ED, or is seen after radical prostatectomy or pelvic surgery) The SHIM gives a severity index, a common vocabulary, and has supplanted vascular testing in many cases. The SHIM, however, is not predictive of outcome.

The Androgen Deficiency in the Aging Male (ADAM) questionnaire, while not sensitive for hypogonadism, asks questions that are pertinent to the hypogonadal state.[124] It is not recommended by the new Endocrine Guidelines to be used for overall screening, due to lack of specificity.[57]

The physical examination for evaluation of male sexual dysfunction in primary care is delineated in **Box 3**. This directed examination is relatively straightforward. **Box 4** describes the laboratory work that is suggested for male sexual dysfunctions as a whole, and that which is optional for the patient.

SUMMARY

Men's health, now as an office evaluation in primary care, requires a thorough understanding of the implications of male sexual dysfunctions, hypogonadism, and cardiometabolic risk stratification and aggressive risk management. The paradigm of the men's health office visit in primary care is the recognition and assessment of male sexual dysfunction, specifically ED, and its value as a signal of overall cardiometabolic health, including the emerging evidence linking low testosterone and metabolic syndrome. A body of evidence from basic science and clinical research is rapidly emerging to make the compelling argument for endothelial cell dysfunction as a central etiologic factor in the development of CVD and other systemic vascular diseases (stroke or vascular claudication). Indeed, ED may now be thought of as a harbinger of cardiovascular clinical events in some men, with an association of risk for an incident cardiovascular event similar to that of current smoking or a family history of myocardial infarction.

This awareness of ED as a barometer for vascular health and occult CVD represents a unique opportunity for primary prevention of vascular disease in all men. However, for this to occur, both urologist and primary care physician must work together to collectively identify and treat modifiable risk factors. It is prudent for the urologist to note these risk factors in those men who present for sexual dysfunction, and ensure that they are evaluated fully by a knowledgable primary care physician.

The optimal relationship between primary care physician and urologist would involve a collaborative desire and communication to comanage those issues vital to men's health: the enlarged prostate; prostate cancer detection and prevention; hormonal replacement therapy; postprostatectomy penile rehabilitation; LUTS; sexual dysfunctions of all types; and finally, cardiovascular risk evaluation and reduction in men with ED. To paraphrase Richardson and Vinik: "a flagging penis should raise the red flag of warning to evaluate the patient for arterial disease elsewhere."[125] This collaborative or shared care model for male sexual dysfunction is being explored in Europe, and now in the United States.

REFERENCES

1. Fontanarosa PB. Theme issue on men's health: call for papers. JAMA 2006;295:440–1.
2. Agency for Healthcare Research and Quality. AHRQ Publication No. 06-0018. December, 2005.
3. Chandra A, Martinez GM, Mosher WD, et al. Fertility, family planning, and reproductive health of U.S. women: Data from the 2002 National Survey of Family Growth. National Center for Health Statistics. Vital Health Stat 2005;23(25):1–160.
4. Kung HC, Hoyert DL, Xu J, et al. National vital statistics report. Vol. 56, Number 10. Deaths: final data for 2005.
5. Penson D, Kreiger JN. Men's health. Are we missing the big picture? J Gen Intern Med 2001; 16:717–71.
6. Barton A. Men's health: a cause for concern. Nurs Stand 2000;15(10):47–52.
7. Courtenay WH. Constructions of masculinity and their influence on men's well being: a theory of gender and health. Soc Sci Med 2000;50:1385–401.
8. Rose I, Kim MT, Dennison CR, et al. The contexts of adherence for African Americans with high blood pressure. J Adv Nurs 2000;32:587–94.
9. Plascencia A, Ostfield AM, Gruber SB. Effects of sex on differences in awareness, treatment, and control of blood pressure. Am J Prev Med 1988;4: 315–26.
10. Sandman D, Simantov E, An C. Out of touch: American men and the health care system.

Commonwealth fund men's and women's health survey findings. Commonwealth Fund; 2000

11. Thompson IM, Tangen CM, Goodman PJ, et al. Erectile dysfunction and subsequent cardiovascular disease. JAMA 2005;294(23):2996–3002.

12. Krane RJ, Goldstein I, Saenz de Tejada I. Impotence. N Engl J Med 1989;321:1648–59.

13. Rosen RC, Leiblum SR. Erectile disorders: an overview of historical trends and clinical perspectives. In: Rosen RC, Leiblum SR, editors. Erectile disorders: assessment and treatment. New York: Guilford; 1992. p. 3–26.

14. NIH Consensus Conference. Impotence. NIH consensus development panel on impotence. JAMA 1993;270(1):83–90.

15. Feldman HA, Goldstein I, Hatzichristou DG, et al. Impotence and its medical and psychosocial correlates: results of the Massachusetts Male Aging Study. J Urol 1994;151:54.

16. Laumann E, Paik A, Rosen RC. Sexual dysfunction in the United States: prevalence and predictors. JAMA 1999;281(6):537–44.

17. Saigal CS, Wessels H, Pace J, et al. Predictors and prevalence of erectile dysfunction in a racially diverse population. Arch Intern Med 2006;166:207–12.

18. Seftel AD, Sun P, Swindle R. The prevalence of hypertension, hyperlipidemia, diabetes mellitus and depression in men with erectile dysfunction. J Urol 2004;171(6 Pt 1):2341–5.

19. Min JK, Williams KA, Okwuosa TM, et al. Prediction of coronary heart disease by erectile dysfunction in men referred for nuclear stress testing. Arch Intern Med 2006;166:201–6.

20. Grover SA, Lowensteyn I, Kaouache M, et al. The prevalence of erectile dysfunction in the primary care setting. Arch Intern Med 2006;166:213–9.

21. Montorsi P, Ravagnani PM, Galli S, et al. Association between erectile dysfunction and coronary artery disease. Role of coronary clinical presentation and extent of coronary vessels involvement: the COBRA trial. Eur Heart J 2006;27(22):2632–9.

22. Azadzoi KM, Goldstein I. Erectile dysfunction due to atherosclerotic vascular disease: the development of an animal model. J Urol 1992;147:1675–81.

23. Montorsi P, Ravagnani P, Galli S, et al. Association between erectile dysfunction and coronary artery disease: matching the right target with the right test in the right patient. Eur Urol 2006;50:721–31.

24. Jackson G, Rosen RC, Kloner RA, et al. The second Princeton consensus on sexual dysfunction and cardiac risk: new guidelines for sexual medicine. J Sex Med 2006;3:28–36.

25. Gazzaruso C, Solerte SB, Pujia A, et al. Erectile dysfunction as a predictor of cardiovascular events and death in diabetic patients with angiographically proven asymptomatic coronary artery disease: a potential protective role for statins and 5-phosphodiesterase inhibitors. J Am Coll Cardiol 2008;51(21):2040–4.

26. Ma RC, So WY, Yang X, et al. Erectile dysfunction predicts coronary artery disease in type 2 diabetics. J Am Coll Cardiol 2008;51(21):2045–50.

27. Hacket G. The burden and extent of comorbid conditions in patients with erectile dysfunction. Int J Clin Pract 2009;63(8):1205–13.

28. Inman BA, Sauver JL, Jacobson DJ, et al. A population-based longitudinal study of erectile dysfunction and future coronary artery disease. Mayo Clin Proc 2009;84(2):108–13.

29. Mykletun A, Dahl AA, O'Leary MP, et al. Assessment of male sexual function by the Brief Sexual Function Inventory. BJU Int 2006;97:316–23.

30. Miner M, Kuritzky L. Erectile dysfunction: a sentinel marker for cardiovascular disease in primary care. Cleve Clin J Med 2007;74:S30–7.

31. Montorsi P, Montorsi F, Schulman CC. Is erectile dysfunction the "tip of the iceberg" of a systemic vascular disorder? [editorial]. Eur Urol 2003;44(3): 352–4.

32. O'Rourke MF, Hashimoto J. Mechanical factors in arterial aging: a clinical perspective. J Am Coll Cardiol 2007;50:1–13.

33. Caretta N, Palego P, Ferlin A, et al. Resumption of spontaneous erections in selected patients affected by erectile dysfunction and various degrees of carotid wall alteration: role of tadalafil. Eur Urol 2005;48:326–31.

34. Bohm M, Baumhakel M, Teo K, et al, for the ONTARGET/TRANSCEND Erectile Dysfunction Substudy Investigators. Erectile dysfunction predicts events in high-risk patients receiving telmisatan, ramipril, or both. Circulation 2010;121:1439–46.

35. Billups KL, Blank AJ, Padma-Nathan H, et al. Erectile dysfunction is a marker for cardiovascular disease: results of the Minority Health Institute Expert Advisory Panel. J Sex Med 2005;2:40–52.

36. Alderman EL, Corley SD, Fisher LD, et al. Five-year angiographic follow-up of factors associated with progression of coronary artery disease in the Coronary Artery Surgery Study (CASS). J Am Coll Cardiol 1993;22:1141–54.

37. Lloyd-Jones DM, Leip EP, Larson MG, et al. Prediction of lifetime risk for cardiovascular disease by risk factor burden at 50 years of age. Circulation 2006;113:791–8.

38. Kostis JB, Jackson G, Rosen R, et al. Sexual dysfunction and cardiac risk (the Second Princeton Consensus Conference). Am J Cardiol 2005;96(2): 313–21.

39. Laumann EO, Nicolosi A, Glasser DB, et al. Sexual problems among women and men aged 40-80 y: prevalence and correlates identified in the global study of sexual attitudes and behaviors. Int J Impot Res 2005;17:39–57.

40. de Boer BJ, Bots ML, Lycklama A, et al. The prevalence of bother, acceptance, and need for help in men with erectile dysfunction. J Sex Med 2005;2: 445–50.

41. Korenman SG. New insights into erectile dysfunction: a practical approach. Am J Med 1998;105: 135–44.

42. Fugl-Meyer AR, Lodnert G, Branholm IB, et al. On life satisfaction in male erectile dysfunction. Int J Impot Res 1997;9:141–8.

43. Rosen RC, Cappelleri JC, Smith MD, et al. Development and evaluation of an abridged, 5-item version of the International Index of Erectile Function (IIEF-5) as a diagnostic tool for erectile dysfunction. Int J Impot Res 1999;11(6):319–26.

44. Gades NM, Nehra A, Jacobson DJ, et al. Association between smoking and erectile dysfunction: a population-based study. Am J Epidemiol 2005; 161(4):346–51.

45. Bacon CG, Mittleman MA, Kawachi I, et al. A prospective study of risk factors for erectile dysfunction. J Urol 2006;176(1):217–21.

46. Hatzichristou D, Rosen RC, Broderick G, et al. Clinical evaluation and management strategy for sexual dysfunction in men and women. J Sex Med 2004;1(1):49–57.

47. Wang C, Nieschlag E, Swerdloff RS, et al. ISA, ISSAM, EAU, EAA and ASA recommendations: investigation, treatment and monitoring of late-onset hypogonadism in males. Aging Male 2009; 12:5–12.

48. Seftel AD. Male hypogonadism. Part I: epidemiology of hypogonadism. Int J Impot Res 2006; 18(2):115–20.

49. Rhoden EL, Morgentaler A. Risks of testosterone-replacement therapy and recommendations for monitoring. N Engl J Med 2004;350:482–92.

50. Harman SM, Metter EJ, Tobin JD, et al. Longitudinal effects of aging on serum total and free testosterone levels in healthy men. Baltimore Longitudinal Study of Aging. J Clin Endocrinol Metab 2001;86: 724–31.

51. Morley JE, Kaiser FE, Perry HM III, et al. Longitudinal changes in testosterone, luteinizing hormone, and follicle-stimulating hormone in healthy older men. Metabolism 1997;46:410–3.

52. Mulligan T, Frick MF, Zuraw QC, et al. Prevalence of hypogonadism in males aged at least 45 years: the HIM study. Int J Clin Pract 2006;60(7):762–9.

53. Snyder PJ. Effects of age on testicular function and consequences of testosterone treatment. J Clin Endocrinol Metab 2001;86:2369–72.

54. Vermeulen A. Androgen replacement therapy in the aging male: a critical evaluation. J Clin Endocrinol Metab 2001;86:2380–90.

55. Bremner WJ, Vitiello MV, Prinz PN. Loss of circadian rhythmicity in blood testosterone levels with aging in normal men. J Clin Endocrinol Metab 1983;56:1278–81.

56. Bhasin S, Cunningham GR, Hayes F, et al. Testosterone therapy in adult men with androgen deficiency syndromes: An Endocrine Society Clinical Practice Guideline. J Clin Endocrinol Metab 2006; 91:1995–2010.

57. Bhasin S, Cunningham GR, Hayes FJ, et al. Testosterone therapy in men with androgen deficiency syndromes: an endocrine society clinical practice guideline. J Clin Endocrinol Metab 2010;95: 2536–59.

58. Institute of Medicine. Testosterone and aging: clinical research directions. Committee on assessing the need for clinical trials of testosterone replacement therapy. Washington, DC: National Academics Press; 2003.

59. Shames D, Gassman A, Handelsman H. Commentary: guideline for male testosterone therapy: a regulatory perspective. J Clin Endocrinol Metab 2007;92(2):414–5.

60. Makhsida N, Shah J, Yan G, et al. Hypogonadism and metabolic syndrome: implications for testosterone therapy. J Urol 2005;174:827–34.

61. Dhindsa S, Prabhakar S, Sethi M, et al. Frequent occurrence of hypogonadotropic hypogonadism in type 2 diabetes. J Clin Endocrinol Metab 2004; 89:5462–8.

62. Corrales JJ, Burgo RM, Garca-Berrocal B, et al. Partial androgen deficiency in aging type 2 diabetic men and its relationship to glycemic control. Metabolism 2004;53:666–72.

63. Ding EL, Song Y, Malik VS, et al. Sex differences of endogenous sex hormones and risk of type 2 diabetes: a systematic review and meta-analysis. JAMA 2006;295:1288–99.

64. Pitteloud N, Mootha VK, Dwyer AA, et al. Relationship between testosterone levels, insulin sensitivity, and mitochondrial function in men. Diabetes Care 2005;28:1636–42.

65. Smith MR, Lee H, Nathan DM. Insulin sensitivity during combined androgen blockade for prostate cancer. J Clin Endocrinol Metab 2006;91:1305–8.

66. Kalme T, Seppala M, Qiao Q, et al. Sex hormone-binding globulin and insulin-like growth factor-binding protein-1 as indicators of metabolic syndrome, cardiovascular risk, and mortality in elderly men. J Clin Endocrinol Metab 2005;90:1550–6.

67. Fukui M, Kitagawa Y, Nakamura N, et al. Association between serum testosterone concentration and carotid atherosclerosis in men with type 2 diabetes. Diabetes Care 2003;26:1869–73.

68. Betancourt-Albrecht M, Cunningham GR. Hypogonadism and diabetes. Int J Impot Res 2003; 15(Suppl 4):S14–20.

69. Tsai EC, Matsumoto AM, Fujimoto WY, et al. Association of bioavailable, free, and total testosterone

with insulin resistance: influence of sex hormone-binding globulin and body fat. Diabetes Care 2004;27:861–8.

70. Laaksonen DE, Niskanen L, Punnonen K, et al. Sex hormones, inflammation and the metabolic syndrome: a population-based study. Eur J Endocrinol 2003;149:601–8.

71. Laaksonen DE, Niskanen L, Punnonen K, et al. Testosterone and sex hormone-binding globulin predict the metabolic syndrome and diabetes in middle-aged men. Diabetes Care 2004;27:1036–41.

72. Laaksonen DE, Niskanen L, Punnonen K, et al. The metabolic syndrome and smoking in relation to hypogonadism in middle-aged men: a prospective cohort study. J Clin Endocrinol Metab 2005;90:712–9.

73. Mokdad AH, Ford ES, Bowman BA, et al. Prevalence of obesity, diabetes, and obesity-related health risk factors, 2001. JAMA 2003;289:76–9.

74. Sullivan PW, Morrato EH, Ghushchyan V, et al. Obesity, inactivity, and the prevalence of diabetes and diabetes-related cardiovascular comorbidities in the U.S., 2000-2002. Diabetes Care 2005;28:1599–603.

75. Ford ES. Prevalence of the metabolic syndrome defined by the International Diabetes Federation among adults in the U.S. Diabetes Care 2005;28:2745–9.

76. Niskanen L, Laaksonen DE, Punnonen K, et al. Changes in sex hormone-binding globulin and testosterone during weight loss and weight maintenance in abdominally obese men with the metabolic syndrome. Diabetes Obes Metab 2004;6:208–15.

77. Boyanov MA, Boneva Z, Christov VG. Testosterone supplementation in men with type 2 diabetes, visceral obesity and partial androgen deficiency. Aging Male 2003;6:1–7.

78. Steidle C, Schwartz S, Jacoby K, et al. the North American AA2500 T Gel Study Group. AA2500 testosterone gel normalizes androgen levels in aging males with improvements in body composition and sexual function. J Clin Endocrinol Metab 2003;88:2673–81.

79. Liu PY, Yee B, Wishart SM, et al. The short-term effects of high-dose testosterone on sleep, breathing, and function in older men. J Clin Endocrinol Metab 2003;88:3605–13.

80. Malkin CJ, Pugh PJ, Jones RD, et al. The effect of testosterone replacement on endogenous inflammatory cytokines and lipid profiles in hypogonadal men. J Clin Endocrinol Metab 2004;89:3313–8.

81. Kapoor D, Goodwin E, Channer KS, et al. Testosterone replacement therapy improves insulin resistance, glycaemic control, visceral adiposity and hypercholesterolaemia in hypogonadal men with

type 2 diabetes. Eur J Endocrinol 2006;154:899–906.

82. Pagotto U, Gambineri A, Pelusi C, et al. Testosterone replacement therapy restores normal ghrelin in hypogonadal men. J Clin Endocrinol Metab 2003;88:4139–43.

83. Yeap BB, Chubb SA, Hyde Z, et al. Lower serum testosterone is independently associated with insulin resistance in non-diabetic older men: the Health In Men Study. Eur J Endocrinol 2009;161:591–8.

84. Stellato RK, Feldman HA, Hamdy O, et al. Testosterone, sex hormone-binding globulin, and the development of type 2 diabetes in middle-aged men: prospective results from the Massachusetts Male Aging Study. Diabetes Care 2000;23:490–4.

85. Selvin E, Feinleib M, Zhang L, et al. Androgens and diabetes in men. Diabetes Care 2007;30:234–8.

86. Pitteloud N, Hardin M, Dwyer AA, et al. Increasing insulin resistance is associated with a decrease in Leydig cell testosterone secretion in men. J Clin Endocrinol Metab 2005;90:2636–41.

87. Oh JY, Barrett-Connor E, Wedick NM, et al. Rancho Bernardo Study. Endogenous sex hormones and the development of type 2 diabetes in older men and women; the Rancho Bernardo study. Diabetes Care 2002;25:55–60.

88. Kupelian V, Shabsigh R, Araujo AB, et al. Erectile dysfunction as a predictor of the metabolic syndrome in aging men: results from the Massachusetts Male Aging Study. J Urol 2006;176:201–6.

89. Esposito K, Giugliano F, Di Palo C, et al. Effect of lifestyle changes on erectile dysfunction in obese men: a randomized controlled trial. JAMA 2004;291(24):2978–84.

90. Traish AM, Guay A, Feeley R, et al. The dark side of testosterone deficiency: I. Metabolic syndrome and erectile dysfunction. J Androl 2009;30:10–22.

91. Traish AM, Saad F, Guay A. The dark side of testosterone deficiency: II. Type 2 diabetes and insulin resistance. J Androl 2009;30:23–32.

92. Traish AM, Saad F, Feeley RJ, et al. The dark side of testosterone deficiency: III. Cardiovascular disease. J Androl 2009;30:477–94.

93. Hak AE, Witteman JC, de Jong FH, et al. Low levels of endogenous androgens increase the risk of atherosclerosis in elderly men: the Rotterdam Study. J Clin Endocrinol Metab 2002;87:3632–9.

94. Phillips G, Pinkernell B, Jing T. The association of hypotestosteronemia with coronary artery disease in men. Arterioscler Thromb 1994;14:701–6.

95. Srinivas-Shankar U, Roberts SA, Connolly MJ, et al. Effects of testosterone on muscle strength, physical function, body composition, and quality of life in intermediate-frail and frail elderly men: a randomized, double-blind, placebo-controlled study. J Clin Endocrinol Metab 2010;95:639–50.

96. van Pottelbergh I, Braeckman L, De Bacquer D, et al. Potential contribution of testosterone and estradiol in the determination of cholesterol and lipoprotein profile in healthy middle-aged men. Atherosclerosis 2003;166:95–102.

97. Makinen JI, Perheentupa A, Irjala K, et al. Endogenous testosterone and serum lipids in middle-aged men. Atherosclerosis 2008;197:688–93.

98. Makinen J, Jarvisalo M, Pollanen P, et al. Increased carotid atherosclerosis in andropausal middle-aged men. J Am Coll Cardiol 2005;45:1603–8.

99. Simon D, Charles MA, Nahoul K, et al. Association between plasma testosterone and cardiovascular risk factors in healthy adult men: the Telecom study. J Clin Endocrinol Metab 1997;82:682–5.

100. Allan CA, Strauss BJ, Burger HG, et al. Testosterone therapy prevents gain in visceral adipose tissue and loss of skeletal muscle in nonobese aging men. J Clin Endocrinol Metab 2008;93:139–46.

101. Basaria S, Muller DC, Carducci MA, et al. Hyperglycemia and insulin resistance in men with prostate carcinoma who receive androgen-deprivation therapy. Cancer 2006;106:581–8.

102. Haidar A, Yassin A, Saad F, et al. Effects of androgen deprivation on glycaemic control and on cardiovascular biochemical risk factors in men with advanced prostate cancer with diabetes. Aging Male 2007;10:189–96.

103. Yialamas MA, Dwyer AA, Hanley E, et al. Acute sex steroid withdrawal reduces insulin sensitivity in healthy men with idiopathic hypogonadotropic hypogonadism. J Clin Endocrinol Metab 2007;92:4254–9.

104. Traish AM, Feeley RJ, Guay A. Mechanisms of obesity and related pathologies: androgen deficiency and endothelial dysfunction may be the link between obesity and erectile dysfunction. FEBS J 2009;276:5755–67.

105. Fukui M, Kitagawa Y, Ose H, et al. Role of endogenous androgen against insulin resistance and atherosclerosis in men with type 2 diabetes. Curr Diabetes Rev 2007;3:25–31.

106. Akishita M, Hashimoto M, Ohike Y, et al. Low testosterone level is an independent determinant of endothelial dysfunction in men. Hypertens Res 2007;30:1029–34.

107. Akishita M, Hashimoto M, Ohike Y, et al. Low testosterone level as a predictor of cardiovascular events in Japanese men with coronary risk factors. Atherosclerosis 2009;210:232–6.

108. Nettleship JE, Pugh PJ, Channer KS, et al. Inverse relationship between serum levels of interleukin-1beta and testosterone in men with stable coronary artery disease. Horm Metab Res 2007;39:366–71.

109. Traish AM, Abdou R, Kypreos KE. Androgen deficiency and atherosclerosis: the lipid link. Vascul Pharmacol 2009;51:303–13.

110. Allan CA, McLachan RI. Age related changes in testosterone and the role of replacement therapy in older men. Clin Endocrinol 2004;60:653–70.

111. Wang C, Swerdloff RS, Iranmanesh A, et al. Transdermal testosterone gel improves sexual function, mood, muscle strength, and body composition parameters in hypogonadal men. J Clin Endocrinol Metab 2000;85:2839–53.

112. Heufelder AE, Saad F, Bunck MC, et al. Fifty-two-week treatment with diet and exercise plus transdermal testosterone reverses the metabolic syndrome and improves glycemic control in men with newly diagnosed type 2 diabetes and subnormal plasma testosterone. J Androl 2009;30:726–33.

113. Caminiti G, Volterrani M, Iellamo F, et al. Effect of long-acting testosterone treatment on functional exercise capacity, skeletal muscle performance, insulin resistance, and baroreflex sensitivity in elderly patients with chronic heart failure a double-blind, placebo-controlled, randomized study. J Am Coll Cardiol 2009;54:919–27.

114. Shores MM, Matsumoto AM, Sloan KL, et al. Low serum testosterone and mortality in male veterans. Arch Intern Med 2006;166:1660–5.

115. Khaw KT, Dowsett M, Folkerd E, et al. Endogenous testosterone and mortality due to all causes, cardiovascular disease, and cancer in men: European Prospective Investigation Into Cancer in Norfolk (EPIC-Norfolk) Prospective Population Study. Circulation 2007;116:2694–701.

116. Laughlin GA, Barrett-Connor E, Bergstrom J. Low serum testosterone and mortality in older men. J Clin Endocrinol Metab 2008;93:68–75.

117. Basaria S, Coviello AD, Travison TG, et al. Adverse events associated with testosterone administration. N Engl J Med 2010;363(2):109–22.

118. Lorenzo C, Williams K, Hunt KJ, et al. The National Cholesterol Education program—Adult Treatment Panel III, International Diabetes Federation, and World Health Organization definitions of the metabolic syndrome as predictors of incident cardiovascular disease and diabetes. Diabetes Care 2007;30:8–13.

119. Esposito K, Giugliano F, Martedi E, et al. High proportions of erectile dysfunction in men with metabolic syndrome. Diabetes Care 2005;28:1201–3.

120. Guembe MJ, Toledo E, Barba J, et al. Association between metabolic syndrome or its components and asymptomatic cardiovascular disease in the RIVANA-study. Atherosclerosis 2010;211(2):612–7.

121. Expert Panel on Detection, Evaluation, and Treatment of High Blood Cholesterol in Adults. Executive

summary of the third report of the National Cholesterol Education Program (NCEP) Expert Panel on Detection, Evaluation and Treatment of High Blood Cholesterol in Adults (Adult Treatment Panel III). JAMA 2001;285:2486–97.

122. Anawalt BD. Guidelines for testosterone therapy for men: how to avoid a mad (T)ea party by getting personal [editorial]. J Clin Endocrinol Metab 2010; 95:2614–7.

123. McLachlan RI. Certainly more guidelines than rules [editorial]. J Clin Endocrinol Metab 2010;95: 2610–3.

124. Morley JE, Charlton E, Patrick P, et al. Validation of a screening questionnaire for androgen deficiency in aging males. Metabolism 2000;49:1239–42.

125. Richardson D, Vinik A. Etiology and treatment of erectile failure in diabetes mellitus. Curr Diab Rep 2002;2:501.

Advocacy in Male Health: A State Society Story

Richard S. Pelman, MD[a,b,*], Deborah A. Johnson, BA[c,d]

KEYWORDS

- Men's health • Prostate cancer screening
- Legislation • Advocacy

How many men have urologists seen who present for evaluation of concerns regarding erectile dysfunction, prostate cancer, vasectomy consultation or evaluation of genital pains, who have no contact with a primary care physician? These men are not referred and are unaware of potential health issues either associated with the condition for which they are seeking care, or they are related to a positive family history for a major disease entity.

Additionally how many referred patients are urologists asked to see for whom the patients' referring physician is unaware of the systemic multiorgan implications of the urological issue being addressed? In both situations the evaluating urologist may have the opportunity to significantly impact the patient's wellbeing. Clearly the male patient who is advised that his difficulties with sexual health lie in multiple system dysfunction is provided with evaluation and treatment that not only address erection issues but may be lifesaving as well. How many patients have returned after such an encounter to say thank you, commenting that had they not been referred on for medical care, would have most likely suffered a stroke or myocardial infarction and considered the identification of underlying obesity, diabetes, hypertension, and coronary artery disease a lifesaving

intervention? Similar is the patient who responded to the suggestion that he have a colonoscopy, and was found to have an early and curable stage of colon cancer.

These are not unique stories to those who practice, yet a pattern of male patients at risk due to lack of entry into the health care system has repeatedly presented itself, and still occurs with regularity.

To improve opportunities for men to recognize the importance of a timely entry into the health care system, The Washington State Urology Society embarked upon a campaign to educate men and their families. Men were felt to be lacking the necessary information in how to take care of themselves, and correction of this knowledge deficit was considered a reasonable remedy. In 1994, The Men's Health Seminar series was developed, and the first seminar was held in the spring of 1995.

A WELL ORGANIZED STATE UROLOGY SOCIETY

Integral to the ability to initiate and carry forth a campaign on male health was a well organized and supported state society. The Washington State Urology Society was established in 1984, with a committed membership and board of

[a] Department of Urology, University of Washington School of Medicine, Box 356510, 1959 NE Pacific, BB-1128, Seattle, WA 98195, USA
[b] Committee on Men's Health, Washington State Urology Society, 914 164th Street SE, #244, Mill Creek, WA 98012, USA
[c] Northwest Chapter, Association for Strategic Planning, 12021 Wilshire Boulevard, #286, Los Angeles, CA 90025, USA
[d] Washington State Urology Society, 914 164th Street SE, #244, Mill Creek, WA 98012, USA
* Corrresponding author. Committee on Men's Health, Washington State Urology Society, 914 164th Street SE, #244, Mill Creek, WA 98012.
E-mail address: rpelman@waurology.com

Urol Clin N Am 39 (2012) 25–31
doi:10.1016/j.ucl.2011.09.009
0094-0143/12/$ – see front matter © 2012 Elsevier Inc. All rights reserved.

directors. The society also benefited from the fact that its leadership included urologists who were active within the American Urological Association, The American Association of Clinical Urologists, and the American Board of Urology.

Most importantly, the leadership of the society was welcoming and nurturing to those newly minted from residency training. This tradition of engagement carries on today and provides for a continued integration of efforts both from rural and suburban, large and small practices, and academic and nonacademic practices.

The Men's Health Seminar Series was thus coordinated throughout the state, with urologists and other medical specialties. A typical presentation would include an introduction by a primary care physician who served as moderator and spoke about how to get the most out of the primary care visit.

Information on diet, cardiac disease/hypertension, colorectal cancer, gastroesophageal reflux disease (GERD), skin cancer detection and prevention, and what men should know about hair loss and baldness was also presented. Urological topics included prostate cancer detection and treatment, benign prostate disease, and impotence. The urological presentations were from various institutions and practices. The benefit to the attendees was a coordinated effort to encourage men to assume a more active role in health care and prevention. The benefit to urology and other specialties was the opportunity to educate the public regarding what strategies and investigations specialty physicians felt were important to the health maintenance of the population, rather than have legislators or other nonphysician groups provide less evidence-based data.

The timing was important, as the national health care climate during that time period was much like the current agenda. Of concern for those in active practice were issues regarding access to specialty care and restrictions on ability to practice. The format of the seminars allowed the public to hear directly from care providers about current care recommendations and what was felt to be current practice standards.

The limiting factors were attendance, which was limited to auditorium capacity, and the fact that most attendees were seniors. The seniors gave tremendous feedback regarding the content of the seminars. One recurring theme was that the seniors wished they had the opportunity to have received the information decades earlier. The benefit from the information provided to the population was felt to be more relevant to the younger man.

Reviewing this information with the dilemma of space constraints and difficulty in reaching younger men, who would be more likely to be at work during the day, or attending the needs of family in the evening, it became clear a different approach was needed. Perhaps the information from the seminars could be developed into a printable guide. Researching available materials regarding men's health yielded surprisingly few satisfactory materials. A book on men's health was available through the American Medical Association (AMA); however, it was very comprehensive, and was a difficult quick read. It appeared to be the type of book that would appeal to an individual who was seeking in-depth information. It was not generally something an average young man would be able to obtain directions for health maintenance from at a glance.

Many other materials suffered from the opposite issues. They contained too little. Pamphlets that suggested a man should get a colon check, watch his weight, eat well, and manage blood pressure, contained very little specific information regarding how to and when undertake care. Additional search of the literature under male health yielded information on sexually transmitted disease (STD) prevention or health-specific recommendations regarding sexual health. The report of the Commonwealth Fund[1] was one of the few publications to report on male health disparity. Additionally, articles by Will Courtney[2] discussed the male tendency to defer care and intervention due to male enculturation. It was clear that more was needed in terms of information on general health maintenance for men.

The Washington State Urology Society executive committee agreed to move ahead with the development of its own booklet. The executive committee felt that the society could provide the necessary information for what men would require, or need to learn and do to enter into appropriate health care maintenance. A Guide to Men's Health was developed as an appropriate tool, with sufficient information for the public to realize the care associated with and health strategies involved in male health maintenance.

Authors were sought from the group of presenting physicians of the seminar series. Each presenter was tasked with writing up his or her presentation for a printed format. The goal was to provide sufficient information for the population to understand the why, what, and when of initiating health care. The idea of a male health maintenance manual synched nicely with what was felt to be adequate information without being overly burdensome to read. The Guide to Men's Health (**Fig. 1**) was printed through an unrestricted educational grant from Bayer Pharmaceuticals (Wayne, NJ, USA) in 2003.

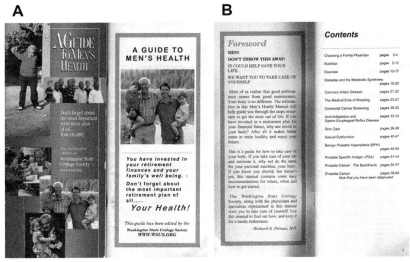

Fig. 1. (*A, B*) The Washington State Urology Society's guide to men's health. (*Courtesy of* the Washington State Urological Society, Mill Creek, WA; with permission.)

Distribution of the printed guide was undertaken with the cooperation of human resource directors of various national and international corporations based in Washington State.

During one such discussion the question was raised: "How do we know a guy who has read it will make an appointment?" Clearly knowledge deficit was only partially responsible for the deficit in male attendance to care. To better answer that question, a collaboration with the Department of Anthropology at the University of Washington was undertaken to further elucidate male health. The pilot study designed to help in developing further data in this regard was by Dr Katherine O'Connor and her team.[3]

Distribution of the printed guide certainly allowed for a greater number of men to access information; however, the opportunity to engage the male population required even a broader reach. Fortunately, the Internet allowed for electronic posting of the guide and the placement of not only the printed Guide to Men's Health, but the posting of video chapters as well. Both versions, as well a Guide to Women's Health, are available at the Web site for the Washington State Urology Society, www.wsus.org.

The video chapters have been well received and have allowed for far greater access to information on male health than the society's first seminars.

ADVOCACY CREATES MORE ADVOCACY

In the Washington State Urology Society's efforts to promote the guide and the men's health agenda, opportunities to meet and engage various other organizations presented collaborations that became beneficial to male health. The experience of promoting the Guide to Men's Health along with the Washington State Urology Society's male health campaign brought together groups that had previously been unaware of each other's efforts. These local organization members were happy to see urologists active in public advocacy on behalf of men. The collaboration with physician champions was helpful in uniting an effort toward promoting the common goal of improved communication toward male health awareness and the importance of pursuing legislative remedies to protect a man's ability to receive appropriate testing as recommended by his health care practitioner. Prostate-specific antigen (PSA) was not routinely being covered by all insurance plans, and in some instances letters from the treating health care professional were required along with supporting documentation with denial still occurring after review.

The relationships developed through the combined advocacy of groups coming together, along with unified acceptance by all parties that prostate cancer detection should be available to all men in Washington State led to a successful legislative campaign. The legislative campaign in the Washington capitol, Olympia, would not have been successful without someone to coordinate the effort. Fortunately, the Washington State Urology Society benefited from a well organized, energetic, and knowledgeable executive director, Debi Johnson, who led the initiative through all the steps and hearings necessary for passage. The process from proposed legislation to passage would not have occurred if Johnson and other committed individuals had not personally guided the bill through the many stages to passage. The ability to band groups together with a common goal allowed legislators to see and hear from not only physician advocates but public advocates as well.

The successful passage of a mandate such as SB 6188 (2006 prostate cancer screening) during a short legislative session in one of the most highly mandated states in the country did not happen overnight. The process took approximately 18 months to complete.

Step 1

Step 1 was identification of an advocacy need that could be translated into a parity bill with a minimal fiscal note. The coverage for prostate cancer screening varied among insurance plans at the time and often involved significant time spent by medical practices to verify benefits for their patients. High-risk patients were receiving their first prostate cancer screen at age 50 and were sometimes diagnosed with late-state disease. This was resulting in increased mortality rates and higher health care costs related to treating these patients. This was frustrating to both the prostate cancer survivor community as well as urologists, knowing prostate cancer is often treatable if diagnosed early. After becoming more informed about the current mammography legislation, Deborah A. Johnson decided there was a need for parity legislation to bring about similar access to prostate cancer screening as there was for breast cancer screening.

Step 2

Through informal interviews with urologists and prostate cancer survivors, it was decided the legislation had to address four critical elements. First, the decision as to whether to screen someone for prostate cancer would no longer be the decision of health insurers. The decision needed to be put back in the hands of medical professionals. Second, the timing of prostate cancer screenings needed to be coordinated by the medical professionals. Third, there needed to be an increased emphasis on prostate cancer awareness for the high-risk populations. Finally, the legislation had to be timeless and nonspecific to a particular screening method, since there were controversies over best practices.

Step 3

Create a public forum to raise awareness for the advocacy need that incorporated all of the key stakeholders and legislative influencers. These included physicians, leaders of primary patient advocacy groups, local television celebrity, chairperson of

the Senate Healthcare Committee, longstanding member on the Senate Health and Long-term Care Committee. Bipartisanship was the key to having any legislative movement on this effort.

Funding for the public forum and patient outreach event was provided by TAP Pharmaceuticals (now known as Abbott Laboratories; North Chicago, IL, USA). The solicitation for the grant funding started in the fall of 2004, when the strategic vision was created. On July 23, 2005, a program called Safe at Home was added to the Regional Softball USA Tournament. Men aged 50 years and older from around the state of Washington and across the country engaged in tournament play and were given the opportunity for a free screening and participation in prostate cancer awareness education. Screenings challenges were set up between the teams regarding "knowing their scores." Key players in the education forum were:

Physicians (Chris Porter, MD, Washington State Urology Society Men's Health Committee member and cochairman of Virginia Mason Medical Center's Urologic Oncology Division)

"Common Urologic Diseases Every Man should know"
–Title of the Education Forum given by Dr Chris Porter.

Patients (including high-risk populations)

President, Seattle Chapter US Too International
Treasurer, US Too International Corporate
Chair, Prostate Cancer (PCa) Task Force of the Washington CARES about Cancer Partnership
President, Man-to-Man Tacoma Chapter
African American Pediatrician PCa survivor
Local television celebrity and PCa survivor
Founder, Safe-At-Home: Prostate Cancer Awareness Network

Legislators on the Senate Health and Long-term Care Committee participated in the town hall meeting on men's health including prostate cancer, which was incorporated into the Safe-At-Home project. (Senator Karen Keiser [D] and Senator Stephen Johnson [R]). It was important to have them at the town hall and have it televised on the local Public Access Network. The goal for the town hall meeting was to capture on film the commitment by legislators to do something in the next legislative session concerning men's health and prostate cancer. The authors were successful in getting a bipartisan commitment to address the issue in the 2006 legislative session.

Step 4

Capture the dialog

The use of a regional nonprofit digital media company and connections with the Public Access Network allowed all of the lectures and panel discussions during the Safe At Home town hall meeting to be captured digitally. Three- to 5-minute edits were created to enforce legislative commitments made during the educational forum. The prostate cancer screening material presented at the forum was edited and streamlined for a comprehensive reference DVD for the senators.

Step 5

Step 5 involves identifying mentors for the legislative process and coordinating partners.

The American Association for Clinical Urologists (AACU) was used as a mentor in the general legislative process. The AACU provided written testimonials that the Washington State Urology Society executive director submitted during legislative hearings. The Washington State Medical Association's (WSMA) director of public policy assisted with the nuances of the Washington State legislature and provided guidance for overcoming potential objections with specific legislators. Although the WSMA could not support the bill because of its policy concerning mandates, the Washington State Urology Society coordinated with members not to publicly state they were against the bill.

The Washington State Urology Society executive director (independent association management contractor and business development consultant) conducted joint strategy sessions with both the TAP Pharmaceuticals and the National Prostate Cancer Coalition's government affairs representatives. The government affairs representative for TAP Pharmaceuticals provided local government insight concerning key legislative players that expedited the process. He lobbied his connections in the state senate and house. His past personal experience working in the Washington State Legislature was helpful. He worked closely with the Washington Legislative Committee staffers to get the behind the scene communications on the status of the bill and made the Washington State Urology Society aware of Novartis Pharma involvement, which increased exposure for the bill.

The National Prostate Cancer Coalition provided additional written testimonials and press releases. In-person testimonies at the legislative hearing were provided by:

US Too International
Man-To-Man

Prostate Cancer Awareness Network
Virginia Mason Medical Center urologist (also provided awareness pins and was instrumental on conducting the free screenings during the Safe At Home event July 2005)
Executive director for the Washington State Urology Society (also purchased pink/blue family pins to reiterate the parity issue surrounding the bill)
Prostate Net
Washington State Prostate Cancer Coalition
American Cancer Society (also provided PCa awareness pins)
Comprehensive Cancer Control Partnership (provided its endorsement).

Step 6

Step 6 involved drafting proposed legislation that met the criteria.

The authors networked with multiple national organizations to identify the best player to assist with drafting of the legislation. It was important to incorporate a national organization that did not appear to have a perceived set agenda (eg, The American Urological Association [AUA] would have a tendency to look like the legislation had a financial benefit to physicians). The National Prostate Cancer Coalition (now known as "ZERO—The Project to End Prostate Cancer") was chosen to be the best partner for this aspect of the strategy.

Step 7

Step 7 involved identifying legislative champions.

Follow-up to the Safe At Home town hall event took place in the fall of 2005. Both Senators Keiser and Johnson were contacted to sponsor the drafted bill. The senators agreed that Senator Johnson would be the best to sponsor it, since Senator Keiser was the chairwoman of the Health and Long-term Care Committee. The Washington State Urology Society cross-referenced recent state legislative speakers for their annual meetings to identify additional champions for the bill. (Linda Evans Parlette (R) and Mary Skinner (R) [diseased as of February 5, 2009]). Additional champions were identified by cross-referencing the Washington State Urological Society/AACU members with legislators sitting on key committees involved with the passage of the bill.

Decision influencers in the legislative process include

Introduce legislation—Senator Johnson
Schedule bill on Senate Health Care Committee agenda and put it up for executive

session—Senator Keiser, Chairwoman of Senate Healthcare

Pull bill out of Senate Rules Committee—Senator Johnson

Place it on the Senate Floor for vote—Senator Tracey Eide (D), Senate Floor Majority

Schedule bill on House Healthcare Committee agenda and put it up for executive session—Representative Eileen Cody (D), chairwoman of House Healthcare

Appropriations hearing agenda and passage—no champion was identified; solicited support from all members of Appropriations committee

Pull bill out of House Rules—Representative Rodney Tom (R during the 2006 legislation year. He switched to D on March 14, 2006)

Place on the House Floor agenda—Representative Frank Chopp (D)

Sign the bill into law—governor.

Step 8

The Washington State Urological Society executive director coordinated society members to participate.

Men's Health Committee member provided scientific references to state senator introducing legislation.

Men's Health Committee member provided testimony at the Senate Health and Long-Term Care Committee hearing Jan. 9, 2006.

Membership was broken down into legislative districts. Strategic committee members and people influencing the flow of the legislative process were identified.

Washington State Urological Society members communicated at strategic times in the legislative process to their state senators and house representative. (eg, President Jeff Frankel, MD, phoned the chairwoman of the House Healthcare Committee as a constituent requesting her to put the bill up for Executive Session). Phone calls were made, and e-mails and faxes were sent.

Step 9

Constant follow-up was made by the executive director of the Washington State Urology Society. Every action was provided a thank you and follow-up. Legislators were asked advice on how to move the bill further in the process. Every thank you and follow-up included visual reminders of the legislation (eg, the family pin, National Prostate Cancer Coalition (NPCC) wrist bands, PCa awareness pins).

A timeline summary is as follows

November 2005—strategy created and funding requests were drafted

July 23, 2006—Safe-At-Home: A Health Project of Us Too International took place at the Senior Softball USA Western Regional Tournament

August 2006—film editing completed and follow-up with senators

September to November 2006—follow-up with senators on commitment of introducing men's health legislation this session

December 2006—provide draft legislation to senator at his request (NPCC provided); Washington State Urological Society Men's Health Committee member provided PSA supporting documentation; society's executive director provided state-specific statistics concerning PCa

January 2007

3—bill was filed and provided number

9—Senate Healthcare Committee hearing (AACU provided testimony)

26—Voted out of Senate Healthcare Committee

30—substitute bill passed to Senate Rules Committee

February 2007

2—pulled out of Rules

8—Voted out of the senate 42 yeas, 1 nay, 2 absent, 4 excused

10—House Healthcare Committee hearing first reading

17—House Healthcare Committee hearing (included AACU testimony)

21—voted out of Healthcare Committee and referred to Appropriations

23—Appropriations Hearing (included AACU testimony)

24—passed to Rules without appropriation because the $50,000 was not in the House budget although it was in the Senate Budget

28—pulled out of Rules Committee

March 2007

1—voted out of the House with 86 yeas, 12 nays

4—Senate concurred with House amendment to remove appropriation

7—president signed and speaker signed

8—delivered to the governor

30—tentative date for governor signature

Benefits of the legislation include

> Increased informed decision making between physicians and their patients
>
> Physicians able to screen patients for prostate cancer regardless of age if they feel it is medically necessary and have it covered by health insurance
>
> $50,000 placed into the state budget for PCa awareness education; although small, it is viewed as a start in the dialog for future funding needs in this area.

Washington State Urology Society pearls for other state societies include

> Work closely with the AACU on state issues.
>
> Get actively involved in the State Society Network to enhance success rates.
>
> Include strategic legislative representatives to participate at state meetings.
>
> Invite legislators (state and federal) to come to one's practice during the nonsession months.
>
> Keep an ongoing dialog with representatives and senators.
>
> Get networked with the government affairs managers of urology venders such as TAP Pharmaceuticals (now known as Abbott Laboratories; North Chicago, IL, USA) and Novartis (East Hanover, NJ, USA).
>
> Include patient advocacy groups in legislative efforts both within the state and on a federal basis.

REFERENCES

1. Sandman D, Simantov E, An C, et al. Out of touch: American men and the health care system, Commonwealth Fund men's and women's health survey findings, March 2000. Available at: http://www.commonwealthfund.org/Publications/Fund-Reports/2000/Mar/Out-of-Touch–American-Men-and-the health care system. Accessed September 9, 2011.

2. Courtenay WH. Constructions of masculinity and their influence on men's well being: a theory of gender and health. Soc Sci Med 2000;50:1385–401.

3. O'Connor KA, Snipes SA, Goodreau SM, et al. Man up: qualitative findings from The Health Initiatives in Men Study. Presented 86th Annual Meeting Western Section, American Urological Association. Waikoloa (HI), October 24, 2010.

Changes in Male Fertility in the Last Two Decades

Kevin R. Loughlin, MD, MBA

KEYWORDS

- Male fertility • Reproductive technology
- Undescended testicules • Cryptorchidism

There can be no greater proof of the recent advances in male fertility than the awarding of the Nobel Prize in Medicine to Robert G. Edwards in 2010. Since the first "test tube" baby, Louise Brown, was born on July 25, 1978, there have been unbridled advances in the diagnosis and treatment of male infertility. There have now been more than 4 million individuals born using assisted reproductive technologies (ARTs), with approximately 170,000 coming from donated oocytes and embryos. Beyond the groundbreaking work of Edwards, there have been many other significant achievements in the treatment of male infertility in recent decades, which are included in this review.

TIMING OF THE SURGICAL REPAIR OF UNDESCENDED TESTICULES

For many years there has been debate among pediatric urologists regarding the timing of the repair of undescended testicules. A prospective, randomized study by Kollin and colleagues[1] addressed this issue. Patients were randomized to surgery at 9 months (72 patients) or 3 years (83 patients) and testicular volume was measured by ultrasonography at ages 6, 12, 24, 39, and 48 months. The ultrasound volume results demonstrated that surgical treatment at 9 months resulted in partial catch-up of testicular growth until at least age 4 years, indicating that early surgery had a beneficial effect on testicular growth. Although testicular growth per se does not predict ultimate fertility, this study provides at least indirect evidence that earlier orchiopexy may be beneficial.

CRYPTORCHIDISM AND TESTICULAR CANCER

Wood and Elder[2] performed a Medline search to provide recommendations concerning the optimum management of cryptochidsm in relation to the development of testicular cancer. They reported that a relative risk of testicular cancer in a cryptorchid case is 2.75 to 8.0. A relative risk of 2 to 3 occurs in patients who undergo orchiopexy by age 12. Patients who undergo orchiopexy after age 12 are 2 to 6 times as likely to have testicular cancer as those who undergo prepubertal orchiopexy. The investigators further reported that a contralateral, normally descended testis in patients with crytorchidsm carries no increased risk of testis cancer.

CRYPTORCHIDISM AND INTRACYTOPLASMIC SPERM INJECTION

Raman and Schlegel[3] evaluated the results of testicular sperm extraction with intracytoplasmic sperm injection (ICSI) in men with nonobstructive azoospermia associated with cryptorchidism. At their institution, they achieved successful retrieval in 35 of 47 testicular sperm extraction attempts (74%) with fertilization in 214 of 347 metaphase II oocytes (62%). Clinical pregnancies resulted for 16 of 35 cycles (46%) when sperm were retrieved, with ongoing pregnancies or deliveries in 15 of the 35 (43%). The investigators identified testicular volume and age at orchiopexy as independent predictors of sperm retrieval for men with a history of cryptorchidism.

Division of Urology, Brigham and Women's Hospital, 45 Francis Street, Boston, MA 02115, USA
E-mail address: kloughlin@partners.org

Urol Clin N Am 39 (2012) 33–36
doi:10.1016/j.ucl.2011.09.004
0094-0143/12/$ – see front matter © 2012 Published by Elsevier Inc.

OPERATIVE APPROACHES FOR VARICOCELECTOMY

Throughout the years, urologists have debated the relative merits of the various operative approaches for varicocele repair. Al-Said and colleagues[4] conducted a prospective randomized study comparing an open inguinal approach (92 patients), laparoscopic approach (94 patients), and a subinguinal microsurgical approach (112 patients). Operative time was significantly longer in the microscopic group and early postoperative complications were comparable in the 3 groups. There was no significant difference in pregnancy rates at 1 year among the 3 groups. Microsurgical repair was associated with no hydrocele formation, a lower incidence of recurrent varicocele, and better improvement in sperm count and motility.

VARICOLECTOMY AND INTRAUTERINE INSEMINATION SUCCESS RATES

Daitch and colleagues[5] reported on 58 couples who were evaluated for infertility. The women were considered normal and all the men had varicoceles. Twenty-four of the men were left untreated and 34 underwent varicocele repair. Although the semen motility rates were not statistically different between the 2 groups, the pregnancy rate was almost double in the group that underwent varicocele ligation. The investigators speculate that functional factors not measured on routine semen analysis may affect pregnancy rates.

INTRACYTOPLASMIC SPERM INJECTION IN THE UNITED STATES

Jain and Gupta[6] analyzed data on ART reported to the Centers for Disease Control and Prevention to determine trends in the use of ICSI and IVF in the United States. They found that the percentage of IVF cycles with the use of ICSI increased dramatically from 11.0% to 57.5% of IVF cycles from 1995 to 2004. This occurred despite the number of cases of male factor conditions remaining stable during this period, suggesting an increasing use of ICSI for conditions other than male factor infertility.

In a related article, Meacham and colleagues[7] estimated that the total expenditure for treating primary male infertility in 2000 was $17 million. It was anticipated that the cost would continue to escalate because there was increasing use of ARTs. Further discussion regarding the economics of male infertility was provided by Meng and colleagues.[8] They used formal decision analysis to estimate and compare the cost-effectiveness of surgical therapy (varicocele ligation and vasectomy reversal) versus ART. Their data suggested that vasectomy reversal is as cost effective as ART if bilateral vasovasostomy can be performed. If a vasoepididymotomy is required, however, sperm retrieval and injection techniques may be more cost effective due to lower patency rates associated with vasoepididymotomy. Vasectomy reversal is more cost effective if patency rates are greater than 79%. They also found that varicocele repair is more cost effective when the postoperative pregnancy rate is greater than 14% in men with a preoperative total motile sperm count of less than 10 million sperm and greater than 45% in men with greater than 10 million total motile sperm. As health care costs continue to rise, the costs of the treatment of male infertility will come under even closer scrutiny.

PERCUTANEOUS EPIDIDYMAL SPERM ASPIRATIONS

Pasqualotto and colleagues[9] reviewed the efficacy of repeat percutaneous epididymal sperm aspiration (PESA) procedures. Although theirs was a small series of only 20 patients, they reported a 37.5% pregnancy rate in patients who underwent repeat PESA. This experience led them to recommend PESA before proceeding to testicular sperm aspiration or extraction.

In a related article, Marmar and colleagues[10] examined the results of vasovasostomy or vasoepididymotomy after failed PESA. Their intraoperative findings demonstrated minimal trauma to the epididymis secondary to PESA. At the time of surgery, sperm were noted in the vasal fluid in 10 of 16 vasal units and a vasovasostomy was possible on at least 1 side in 7 of 8 patients. Vasoepididymotomy was technically possible when needed. Of the 8 couples, 4 achieved a pregnancy.

DRUG THERAPY FOR IDIOPATHIC MALE INFERTILITY

Kumar and colleagues[11] performed a literature review looking at the evidence of the efficacy of drug therapy in the treatment of idiopathic male infertility. Their review revealed no evidence in support of androgens or gonadotropins for enhancing male fertility and these agents may act as contraceptives. They also found insufficient evidence regarding the role of antiestrogens, aromatase inhibitors, and antioxidants to enhance fertility. Their conclusion was that drug therapy for idiopathic male infertility is at best empirical.

MATERNAL SMOKING AND INFERTILITY OF OFFSPRING

Thorup and colleagues[12] prospectively studied 157 boys ages 1 through 5.9 years who presented with cryptorchidism. At the time of the orchiopexy a testicular biopsy was performed. These investigators found that boys whose mothers had smoked heavily during pregnancy (more than 10 cigarettes/day) throughout the pregnancy had increased risk of bilateral cryptorchidism (52% offspring of smokers and 20% nonsmokers) as well as a decreased number of spermatogonia and gonocytes per tubule cross-section.

SIGNIFICANCE OF TESTICULAR ULTRASOUND FINDINGS IN SEVERE MALE INFERTILITY

Carmignani and colleagues[13] retrospectively reviewed 560 infertile men who underwent testicular ultrasound evaluation. Of these men, 8 (1.4%) showed focal testicular lesions, 2 (.4%) were diagnosed with germ cell tumors and 3 (.05%) with interstitial cell neoplasms. Both germ cell tumors were palpable. The investigators concluded that the risk of undiagnosed malignant tumors in men evaluated for infertility was low.

DIAGNOSIS OF EJACULATORY DUCT OBSTRUCTION

Purohit and coworkers[14] prospectively performed transrectal ultrasound (TRUS) and 3 other tests (duct chromotubation, seminal vesicle aspiration, and seminal vesiculography) to evaluate men with ejaculatory duct obstruction. They found that TRUS findings correlated poorly with other modalities. Obstruction on TRUS was confirmed in only 52%, 48%, and 36% of vesiculography seminal vesicle aspiration and duct chromotubation studies, respectively. The investigators concluded that TRUS alone had poor specificity for ejaculatory duct evaluation and recommended that incorporating dynamic tests into the evaluation of ejaculatory duct obstruction may decrease unnecessary duct resection procedures and improve the success rates of resection procedures when indicated.

UNDERWEAR TYPE AND MALE SUBFERTILITY

For many years there has been an assumption by some patients and clinicians that underwear type, loose fitting versus tight, may affect fertility Munkelwitz and Gilbert[15] undertook a critical analysis to determine if this assumption had any factual basis. They measured the scrotal, core, and skin temperatures in 97 consecutive men presenting for evaluation of clinical subfertility. The cases were categorized as to underwear type and baseline semen parameters were obtained in all patients. In 14 patients (crossover group) underwear type was changed to the alternative type and temperature measurements were repeated.

Mean scrotal temperature was 33.8°C ± 0.8°C and 33.6°C ± 1.1°C in the boxer and brief group, respectively. There were no significant temperature differences between the groups. The investigators concluded that the hyperthermic effect of brief style underwear has been exaggerated and that it is unlikely to have a significant effect on male infertility.

WORLDWIDE TRENDS IN MALE FERTILITY

Whether or not overall sperm counts are decreasing continues to be an area of controversy. In 1992, Carlsen and colleagues[16] reported a significant global decline in sperm density between 1938 and 1990. Swan and colleagues[17] published a subsequent study that demonstrated significant declines in sperm density in the United States and Europe/Australia after controlling for abstinence time, age, percent of men with proved fertility, and sample collection method. These investigators reported declines in sperm density in the United States of approximately 1.5% per year and in Europe/Australia of approximately 3.0% per year. These observations may be due to a variety of factors, including both environmental and dietary factors.

In addition to what seems to be objective declines in sperm density, at least in the Western world, there are also lifestyle changes that have an impact on fertility rates.

The World Fertility Report[18] documented that the average age at the time of first marriage is increasing for both men and women. In addition, the report documents that contraception use and divorce rates have also increased over recent decades. The report documented that between the 1970s and the early years of the twenty-first century, fertility fell worldwide in all but one of the 132 countries or areas for which data were available for both periods.

These observed trends suggest that the diagnosis and management of male infertility is likely to increase. It is therefore imperative that training and research in male infertility continue to be areas of focus for urologists.

REFERENCES

1. Kollin C, Karpe B, Hesser V, et al. Surgical treatment of unilateral undescended testes: testicular growth

after randomization to orchiopexy at age 9 months or 3 years. J Urol 2007;178(4 Pt 2):1589–93.

2. Wood HM, Elder JS. Cryptorchidism and testicular cancer: separating fact from fiction. J Urol 2009; 181(2):452–61.

3. Raman JD, Schlegel PN. Testicular sperm extraction with intracytoplasmic sperm injection is successful for the treatment of non obstructive azoospermia associated with cryptorchidism. J Urol 2003;170(Pt 1): 1287–90.

4. Al-Said S, Al-Naimi A, AL-Ansari A, et al. Varicocelectomy for male infertility: a comparative study of open laparoscopic and microsurgical approaches. J Urol 2008;180(1):266–70.

5. Daitch JA, Badiwy MA, Pasqualotto EB, et al. Varicocelectomy improves intrauterine insemination success rates in men with varicocele. J Urol 2001;165(5): 1510–3.

6. Jain T, Gupta RS. Trends in the use of intracytoplasmic sperm injection in the United States. N Engl J Med 2007;357(3):251–7.

7. Meacham RB, Joyce GF, Wisse M, et al. Male infertility. J Urol 2007;177(6):2058–66.

8. Meng MV, Greene KL, Turek PJ. Surgery or assisted reproduction? A decision analysis of treatment costs in male infertility. J Urol 2005;174(5):1926–31.

9. Pasqualotto FF, Rossi-Ferragut LM, Rocha CC, et al. The efficacy of repeat percutaneous epididymal sperm aspiration procedures. J Urol 2003;169(5):1779–81.

10. Marmar JL, Sharlip I, Goldstein N. Results of vasovasostomy or vasoepididymostomy after failed percutaneous epidudymal sperm aspirations. J Urol 2008;179(4):1506–9.

11. Kumar R, Gautam G, Gupta NP. Drug therapy for idiopathic male infertility: rationale versus evidence. J Urol 2006;176(4 Pt 1):1307–12.

12. Thorup J, Cartes D, Peterson BL. The incidence of bilateral cryptorchidism is increased and the fertility potential is reduced in sons born to mothers who have smoked during pregnancy. J Urol 2006; 176(2):734–7.

13. Carmignani L, Gadda F, Mancini M, et al. Detection of testicular ultrasonographic lesions in severe male infertility. J Urol 2004;172(3):1045–7.

14. Purohit RS, Wu DS, Shinohara K, et al. A prospective comparison of 3 diagnostic methods to evaluate ejaculatory duct obstruction. J Urol 2004;171(1): 232–5.

15. Munkelwitz R, Gilbert BR. Are boxer shorts really better? A critical analysis of the role of underwear type in male subfertility. J Urol 1998; 160(4):1329–33.

16. Carlsen E, Giwercman A, Keiding N, et al. Evidence for decreasing quality of semen during the past 50 years. BMJ 1992;305:609–13.

17. Swan SH, Elkin EP, Fenster L. The question of declining sperm density revisited: an analysis of 101 studies published 1934-1996. Environ Health Perspect 2000;108(10):961–6.

18. World Fertility Report. New York: Population Division Department of Economic and Social Affairs, United Nations; 2007.

Men's Health Initiative of British Columbia: Connecting the Dots

S. Larry Goldenberg, CM, OBC, MD, FRCSC

KEYWORDS

- Men's Health • Prevention • Promotion • Outreach
- Advocacy

OVERVIEW

The health risks associated with men's gender or masculinity have remained largely unproblematic.... Left unquestioned, men's shorter lifespan is often presumed to be natural and inevitable[1]

The women's health lens has become an important aspect of planning in many health care systems.[2] Results have been impressive, with better-targeted policies, sophisticated research programs, and improved clinical services acting together to enhance health outcomes for women. An example from British Columbia, Canada is the British Columbia Center of Excellence for Women's Health, established in the early 1970s to respond to unmet health needs identified by leaders in the women's movement.[3] The center has identified and provided comprehensive health services to women for the past 25 years, but there is no equivalent center for men.

The lens through which men's health is examined will influence how it is understood and advanced. As Courtenay highlights[4]:

Most of what we currently understand about men's health is fragmented and diffuse. It is fragmented by the individual disciplinary lenses through which we view men's health as epidemiologists, health educators, medical anthropologists, nurses and physicians, psychiatrists, ethnographers, psychologists, public health workers, social workers and sociologists. These individual lenses enable us to deeply understand very specific aspects of men's health. However, they also often limit the ways in which we conceptualize and understand men's experiences more broadly.

Men's health has matured over the past 2 to 3 decades, and both Australia and Ireland have developed official federal male health policies.[5,6] In Canada, issues around men's health have captured increasing interest of health professionals, researchers, the media, the lay public, and politicians. However, a lack of partnership and synergy within and between research, practice, and policy contexts has encumbered the advancing of men's health promotion in our country.

The Men's Health Initiative of British Columbia (MHIBC) was officially launched in November, 2009. It is organized as an umbrella, a brand name, and a single point of contact to identify and include multiple academic and community foci of interest and excellence and to catalyze cooperation and partnership. In this way, it will facilitate educational collaboration, broad-spectrum research, the gathering or the production and dissemination of best practices or standards of care, and enable the advocacy of men's health issues at all levels of government. The MHIBC will reach out to men across all

The author has nothing to disclose.
Department of Urologic Sciences, University of British Columbia, Level 6, 2775 Laurel Street, Vancouver, BC, Canada V5Z 1M9
E-mail address: l.gold@ubc.ca

Urol Clin N Am 39 (2012) 37–51
doi:10.1016/j.ucl.2011.09.001
0094-0143/12/$ – see front matter © 2012 Elsevier Inc. All rights reserved.

ages, races, and socioeconomic groups and will apply a male lens to current and future health promotion, awareness, and policy activities. A male gender–approach will benefit spouses Vancouver, British Colimbia, Canada: children and extended families and communities by highlighting key gender-specific biologic, psychological, social, and cultural determinants aiming to achieve the best health care possible for the men of British Columbia.

In an early project of the MHIBC, the author and colleagues performed a review of the gray and white literature to address the complexities of decreased male life expectancy and potential years of life lost. This review resulted in the creation of "A Roadmap to Men's Health: Current status, Research Policy and Practice" (The Roadmap), which is an overview of why men's health matters, what we know, gaps in our knowledge/service delivery, and what new directions we should be taking. The scope of the report includes male-specific conditions (eg, prostate cancer, testis cancer, hypogonadism, and sexual dysfunction) and male-risk conditions (conditions for which being a man represents a significant risk factor regarding incidence, outcome, or mortality [eg, cardiovascular disease, lung cancer, osteoporosis, HIV, and suicide]). These conditions are examined in the framework of the factors that underlie sex and gender differences in health status, including differences in health-related attitudes and behaviors.

Because it is unlikely that biology alone can explain all gender differences, much research is required to examine the interplay, perhaps through epigenomic phenomena, between environment, diet, socio-economics, and biologic manifestations of disease. The author presents some of the findings of this extensive report.

Life Expectancy

Gender, as a key determinant of health, and the experience of being a man in our society both strongly affect our health and how it is managed. Many questions need to be asked and answered on gender-specific and gender-dominant issues affecting all the ages and stages of the male lifespan. In Canada and many countries around the world, a consistent pattern of life expectancy has developed over the past century: men die at an earlier age than women. British Columbia provincial data from 2004 to 2008 indicate that men had a mean life expectancy of 78.9 years, whereas women had a mean life expectancy of 83.3 years, a difference of 4.4 years.[7] Life expectancy data for British Columbia over an extended time period (beginning about 1920) show a steady increase in life expectancy for both genders, with women consistently living longer than men (**Fig. 1**). This gender difference in life expectancy was less than 5 years between 1920 and 1940 and then it increased steadily until 1980 at which time

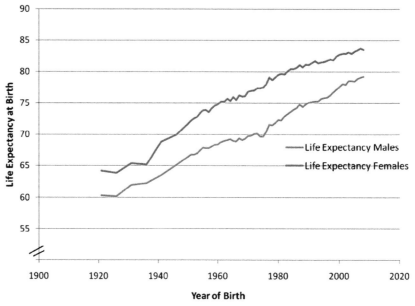

Fig. 1. Life expectancy at birth for British Columbia beginning 1920, showing the increase for both genders and persistent gender gap. (*From* Bilsker D, Goldenberg L, Davison J. A roadmap to men's health: current status, research policy and practice. Vancouver, British Columbia, Canada: Centre for Applied Research in Mental Health and Addiction and The Men's Health Initiative of BC; 2010; with permission.)

women had an almost 8-year advantage in life expectancy. This gender gap decreased just as dramatically between 1980 and the present, returning to a level of just more than 4 years.

There is no clear explanation for this marked fluctuation in relative life expectancy and we cannot predict whether the gender gap in life expectancy will continue to diminish (we simply do not know the factors responsible for changes in the size of this gap). Also, these gender life expectancy differences are fairly consistent across various regions of the province over the past few decades.

Health Expectancy

Beyond length of life, more revealing statistics relate to the age at which a person loses his or her good health (health expectancy) and the numbers of years of life lost because of dying at an early age (potential years of life lost). In general, once men develop a serious health condition, the prognosis is worse than that for women and they are more likely than women to die of it; "in nearly all countries for which data were available, women live longer 'healthier lives' and once sick live from 0.2 years to 7.3 years longer than men in sickness."[6] Such differential health outcomes affect millions of men every year.[9] As one research team has observed: "There is a remarkable discrepancy between the health and survival of the sexes: men are physically stronger and have fewer disabilities, but have substantially higher mortality at all ages compared with women: the so-called male-female health-survival paradox."[10] With an average health expectancy of 65 years, Canadian men may experience 11 or more years of poor health and disability before they die. This figure is even higher in subgroups, such as Native Canadians.

Given this striking discrepancy in life expectancy and the decrease in health expectancy, one would expect to find that men's health has been a high priority for many years, drawing substantial investment of financial and intellectual resources from policymakers and researchers. But in fact, the domain of men's health has been neglected, receiving serious and widespread attention only in the last decade. Through most of the history of health care research and practice, findings of inferior health outcomes for men have been met with a kind of resignation, as though gender disparity in health outcomes were simply an unavoidable feature of the world, something to be accepted rather than addressed.[11]

Clearly, identifying the reasons for differential mortality between men and women, the relative contribution of various causal factors, would enable us to research and develop meaningfully targeted interventions to reduce the gender gap in life expectancy. However, there has been surprisingly little focused research attempting to discover the nature of sex differences associated with the observed life expectancy gap, their causation, and potential remediation.[12,13]

MHIBC: a roadmap to men's health: current status, research, policy and practice

"Having a Y chromosome should not be seen as possessing a self destruct mechanism."[14]

To understand the differences in mortality and other health outcomes between men and women, a framework was developed for this report. This framework included biologic factors (eg, differences in hormone levels between men and women), environmental factors (eg, men being preferentially hired into physically dangerous jobs), and behavioral factors (eg, men taking risks at a high level, being reluctant to adopt positive health behaviors, and not seeking health care services when appropriate). This framework was applied to the leading causes of early male mortality and potential years of life lost.

Data concerning causes of death in British Columbia is available in a report produced by the British Columbia Ministry of Health Planning[15] that shows the incidence of death by various causes in 2002 for men and women. Highlights of the report are presented in **Table 1**, with data clustered by age group: individuals aged 15 to 24 years, 25 to 44 years, 45 to 64 years, and 65 to 84 years. This data table gives us some ideas about the sources of increased mortality of men. For example, we see that unintentional injuries seemed to be a significant source of mortality difference between men and women, with men showing much higher mortality caused by injuries in 2 of the age groups. Cardiovascular disease also presents much higher male mortality. By contrast, mortality caused by cancer is similar for men and women.

This information is useful, but we need something more to make sense of the life-expectancy gap between men and women; we need a statistic that will take into account both the differential rate of mortality *and* the age at which death occurs. A death occurring in one's 20s steals many more years of life than a death occurring in one's 70s. Fortunately, there is an index that is commonly used in epidemiology to take into account these two aspects of mortality. This index is the potential years of life lost (PYLL), which is also known as years of life lost (YLL). The PYLL index indicates the "number of years of life 'lost' when

Table 1
Leading causes of death for BC men and women, 2002

	Men	Women
15–24 y		
Unintentional injuries	105	36
Suicide	34	11
Cancer	9	11
Congenital anomalies	4	7
Disorders of the nervous system	5	3
Other causes	52	27
25–44 y		
Unintentional injuries	231	64
Cancer	98	115
Suicide	110	31
Infections of the nervous system	55	22
Other causes	280	144
45–64 y		
Cancer	943	934
Cardiovascular diseases	546	145
Unintentional injuries	190	53
Liver diseases	113	58
Infectious diseases	94	48
Other causes	786	42
65–84 y		
Cancer	2516	2083
Cardiovascular diseases	1934	1399
Cerebrovascular diseases	492	539
Chronic pulmonary disease	413	351
Diabetes mellitus	290	214
Other causes	1856	1667

a person dies 'prematurely' from any cause, before age 75 – taking the median age in each age group, subtracting from 75, and multiplying by the number of deaths in that age group disaggregated by sex and cause of death."[16] This index is very useful, allowing us to understand the longevity difference between the sexes in how much of the total gap (what proportion of the lost years of life) is attributable to various health conditions.[17] By taking into account not only the rate but also the age of death, the PYLL is a powerful statistic that can help us understand the life expectancy gap in a more profound way, pointing us to key challenges and opportunities for creating change.

It must be noted that the PYLL does not fully measure the potential gain in life expectancy if we were to eliminate specific sources of mortality. This factor is mainly because there are other sources of mortality that would undo some of the gain (eg, preventing a fatal heart attack would not protect that person from other fatal conditions or accidents [competing risks]). There is another statistic for measuring the potential gain from reducing a source of mortality known as potential gains in life expectancy (PGLE). The PGLE, by the elimination of deaths from a particular cause, is the added years of life expectancy for the population if the deaths from that cause were removed or eliminated as a competing risk of death. This type of measurement is based on multiple-decrement life table techniques that properly take into account competing risks of death and the age structure of the population.[18] Unfortunately, available epidemiologic data has mostly not been analyzed in terms of the PGLE. But keeping in mind the problem of competing risks will make us more cautious in projecting the benefit from interventions to reduce a source of male mortality, remembering that another health condition or accident may be waiting its turn to cause death. For example, we might succeed in reducing the likelihood of death from some type of cancer without extending life expectancy (if another condition takes that life around the same age that cancer would have).

In **Fig. 2**, we see the differences between men and women in British Columbia expressed in PYLL, once again organized by age at the time of death. These data are for the year 2006. Not surprisingly, the pattern of mortality changes considerably across the age groups, with motor vehicle accidents accounting for a much higher proportion of PYLL in the younger age groups, whereas cancer becomes the leading cause of death in the 45- to 74-year-old age group. Although not shown here, the pattern among those aged older than 75 years looks quite similar to that found in the 45- to 74-year-old age group. One further step is needed to attain a clear understanding of the differences between men and women in life expectancy: an overall picture of the differences between men and women in years of life lost, across the age groups, ranked in terms of the leading contributors to the life expectancy gap. To obtain this overall picture, the author calculated the difference between PYLL by men and those lost by women, that is, men's PYLL minus women's PYLL across the age groups. In this way, the author was able to identify the 5 sources of mortality contributing most to the life expectancy gap between men and women (**Fig. 3**).

This information provides a novel picture of the life expectancy gap, yielding a different type of

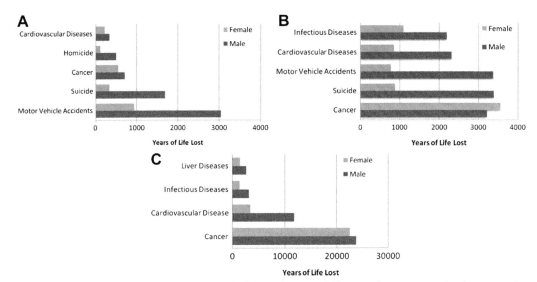

Fig. 2. (*A–C*) Leading causes of potential years of life lost, showing differences between genders by age at time of death. (*From* Bilsker D, Goldenberg L, Davison J. A roadmap to men's health: current status, research policy and practice. Vancouver, British Colimbia, Canada: Centre for Applied Research in Mental Health and Addiction and The Men's Health Initiative of BC; 2010; with permission.)

information from that provided by tables of death rates. Here, we see that the first contributor to the gender gap is cardiovascular disease (CVD), which causes substantial mortality in men at a younger average age than in women. The second greatest contributor to the gender gap is suicide, which affects men more often than women and occurs fairly often in younger age groups. The third greatest contributor to the gender gap is motor vehicle accidents. These accidents are more common and more often fatal in men, occurring relatively often in the younger

age groups. The fourth greatest contributor to the gender gap is infectious disease. Note that the infectious disease accounting for the most years of life lost for men versus women is HIV/AIDS. The fifth greatest contributor to the gender gap is liver disease, with most of the liver disease accounting for years of life lost for men versus women caused by alcohol dependence. This overall picture of the gender gap in life expectancy provides a critically important indication of opportunities for reducing the gap. Each contributor to the gender gap represents an *opportunity*, an

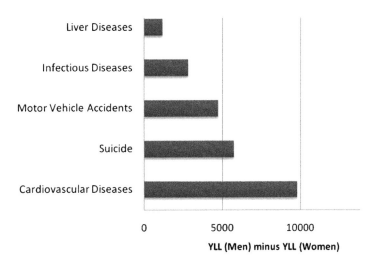

Fig. 3. Five sources of mortality contributing to the excess years of life lost for men versus women. (*From* Bilsker D, Goldenberg L, Davison J. A roadmap to men's health: current status, research policy and practice. Vancouver, British Colimbia, Canada: Centre for Applied Research in Mental Health and Addiction and The Men's Health Initiative of BC; 2010; with permission.)

area in which interventions to improve knowledge or service delivery might make a meaningful improvement in men's health and mortality risk.

Cardiovascular disease It can be seen in **Fig. 4** that the prevalence of heart disease increases more quickly in men than in women, particularly from the 55 to 64 age range onwards. Not surprisingly, this greater prevalence of CVD in men translates into higher rates of CVD-related mortality. **Fig. 5**, also adapted from 2009 Tracking Heart Disease and Stroke in Canada,[19] shows the rates of death caused by CVD between the ages of 25 and 74 years for different age groups. Even more strikingly than in the prevalence graph, we see the greater impact of CVD on men's mortality, beginning in the 55 to 64 age range. As we learned using the PYLL index, both the higher death rate and earlier onset for men contribute to CVD's importance as a source of the average life expectancy gap.

Suicide In Canada, the male suicide rate is about 3 times that of women. **Fig. 6**[7] charts the age- and gender-specific incidence of suicide in Canada, based on data from 2001 to 2005. The chart shows 2 patterns: (1) The male suicide rate increases fairly steadily with age until peaking in the late

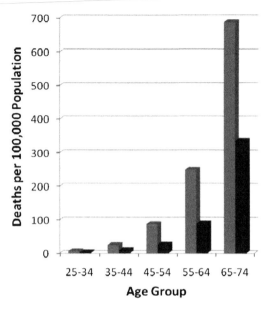

Fig. 5. Rates of death caused by cardiovascular disease in the Canadian population aged 25 to 74 years. (*From* Bilsker D, Goldenberg L, Davison J. A roadmap to men's health: current status, research policy and practice. Vancouver, British Colimbia, Canada: Centre for Applied Research in Mental Health and Addiction and The Men's Health Initiative of BC; 2010; with permission.)

40s, then decreases significantly and increases again in the 80s. (2) Male rates are greater than female rates at all ages and substantially greater across most of the lifespan.

The evident male pattern of peak in suicide rate in the 40s and 50s is surprising in light of multinational data showing one of two patterns: a steady increase in suicide rate with age *or* a peak of suicide in younger age groups.[20,21] However, a change in this suicide pattern may be underway:

Among U.S. white men, middle age has historically been a time of relatively lower risk of completed suicide, compared with elderly men. Yet by 2005, the suicide rate of white men aged 45–49 years was not only higher than the rate for men aged <40 years but also slightly higher than the rate for men aged 70–74 years.... In the past, suicide-prevention efforts have focused most heavily on the groups considered to be most at risk: teens and young adults of both genders as well as elderly white men, whose rates of suicide have historically been the highest in the U.S. Attention and resources dedicated to these subgroups may have increased the awareness and identification of suicide in these populations, perhaps partly because

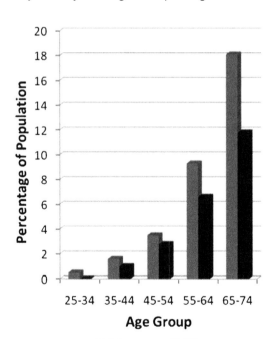

Fig. 4. Self-reported prevalence of cardiovascular disease in the Canadian population, aged 25 to 74, 2007. (*From* Bilsker D, Goldenberg L, Davison J. A roadmap to men's health: current status, research policy and practice. Vancouver, British Colimbia, Canada: Centre for Applied Research in Mental Health and Addiction and The Men's Health Initiative of BC; 2010; with permission.)

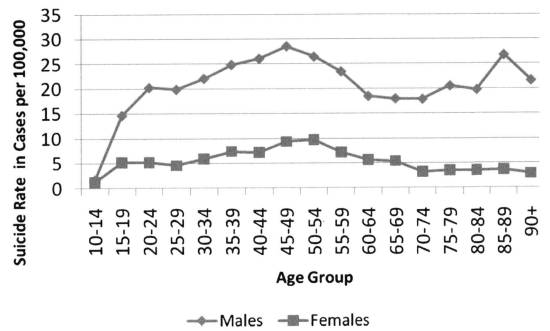

Fig. 6. Median male and female age-specific suicide rates based on Statistics Canada data (2001–2005). (*From* Bilsker D, Goldenberg L, Davison J. A roadmap to men's health: current status, research policy and practice. Vancouver, British Colimbia, Canada: Centre for Applied Research in Mental Health and Addiction and The Men's Health Initiative of BC; 2010; with permission.)

the very young and very old groups are easier to identify or study in settings such as schools or primary care. Suicide in the middle-adult years has not been studied as extensively.[22]

It is apparent that our knowledge of male suicide is lagging behind changes in the age-specific incidence of this source of mortality. Until we understand the underlying reasons for this relative increase in men's dying by suicide in middle age, we will not be able to implement preventative action. Suicide is the second leading source of PYLL by men in comparison with women, reflecting both men's higher rate of suicide and the young age at which many suicide deaths occur (see **Fig. 3**). In Canada, suicide accounts for about 10% of all PYLL for men and in British Columbia, it accounts for about 7%.[7] But the PYLL calculation does not measure the potential gain in life expectancy if we were to eliminate that source of mortality. Men in British Columbia would not live 7% longer on average if we prevented all male suicide. This factor is mainly because of other sources of mortality that would undo some of the gain; preventing an individual's suicide would not protect that person from other health conditions or accidents (competing risks).

In addition to suicide rate, we also need to consider suicide *attempts* to understand the gender difference in suicidal behavior. Although men die by suicide at a higher rate, women have a higher rate of attempting suicide.[23] It should be noted that there is a spectrum of self-harm, ranging from acts of physical self-harm not intended to be suicidal to acts that reflect ambivalence about dying to acts that reflect a clear and settled intention to die. The broad term *deliberate self-harm* (DSH) is used in the research to capture this range of possible actions. As one might expect from the suicide attempt statistics, women show much higher rates of DSH.[24]

Motor vehicle accidents Men are generally more likely to act in physically risky ways when it comes to operating motor vehicles. Considerable evidence shows that young men are more prone than young women to drive at unsafe speeds and in a reckless manner.[25] In British Columbia, the rates of serious injury from motor vehicle accidents (MVA) between 2003 and 2007 declined in both genders but men consistently averaged 12% more injuries than women.

Motor vehicle accidents are among the leading cause of mortality for young men. Because these deaths happen at such a young age, they account for a large proportion of PYLL.[26] As the author has shown, mortality from MVAs is the third leading cause of years of life lost by men in comparison with women (see **Fig. 3**). Mortality rates in British Columbia caused by MVA, by age and gender (for 2007), are shown in **Fig. 7**. The overall pattern of higher male rates is consistent but the gender difference is accentuated, especially in the 16- to 25-year-old age group, accounting for a huge number of life years lost. There is also a higher mortality rate for men aged older than 80 years, but the absolute numbers are small.

HIV/AIDS Based on the incidence of HIV-positive tests, the rate of HIV infection in men is 3 times that in women (**Fig. 8**). Over the time period portrayed in this figure, 1998 to 2007, there does not seem to be any meaningful trend, upwards or downwards, for either gender.

Considering the incidence of a positive HIV test by age, it is evident that the differences between men and women first occur in the 20- to 29-year-old age group (**Fig. 9**). Mortality attributable to HIV infection is shown in **Fig. 10**, presenting the number of deaths attributable to this health condition by year and gender. Clearly, there is a dramatically higher rate of mortality for men than for women. But just as dramatic is a substantial

reduction in HIV-associated mortality. Research performed in Vancouver in the late 1980s and early 1990s found "life expectancy at age 20 years for gay and bisexual men is 8–20 years less than for all men.[27]" Over the last 15 years, male deaths attributable to HIV have declined by 50%. This reduced level of mortality reflects advances in the treatment of HIV infection and a far greater capacity to slow or even halt progression to AIDS. In particular, highly active antiretroviral therapy has proven effective in improving life expectancy of individuals infected with HIV.[28–30]

Alcohol dependence Alcohol dependence (AD) is associated with serious health consequences and increased mortality risk. AD may be defined as the use of alcohol "despite significant areas of dysfunction, evidence of physical dependence, and/or related hardship."[31] **Fig. 11** shows that AD reaches its greatest level of incidence around 18 years of age, is dramatically higher for men than women, and the gender gap declines with age. Given the strikingly high rates of alcohol abuse/dependence among young men, there is clearly an excellent opportunity for programs to prevent

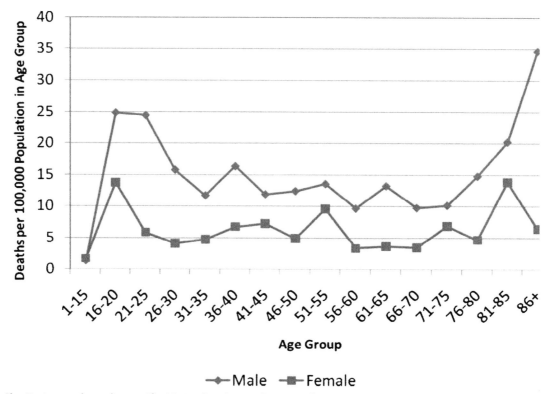

Fig. 7. Age and gender-specific MVA-related mortality rates for 2007 in BC. (*From* Bilsker D, Goldenberg L, Davison J. A roadmap to men's health: current status, research policy and practice. Vancouver, British Colimbia, Canada: Centre for Applied Research in Mental Health and Addiction and The Men's Health Initiative of BC; 2010; with permission.)

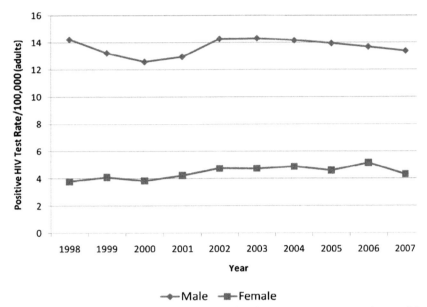

Fig. 8. Incidence of HIV-positive tests in Canada by gender for the years 1998 to 2007. (*From* Bilsker D, Goldenberg L, Davison J. A roadmap to men's health: current status, research policy and practice. Vancouver, British Colimbia, Canada: Centre for Applied Research in Mental Health and Addiction and The Men's Health Initiative of BC; 2010; with permission.)

the onset of this health condition by intervening in high school or before. Indeed, it has been demonstrated that a substantial reduction of alcohol abuse/dependence can be achieved in a cost-effective way through school-based programs.[32]

MHIBC: connecting the dots

What are these dots? They represent the diverse foci of excellence that currently exist throughout the British Columbia health care delivery sectors; government; public health; educational and research

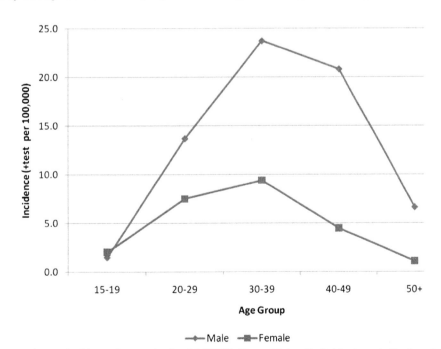

Fig. 9. Age-specific HIV incidence by gender for BC (2007). (*From* Bilsker D, Goldenberg L, Davison J. A roadmap to men's health: current status, research policy and practice. Vancouver, British Colimbia, Canada: Centre for Applied Research in Mental Health and Addiction and The Men's Health Initiative of BC; 2010; with permission.)

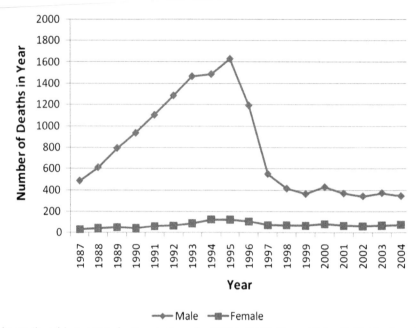

Fig. 10. Deaths attributable to HIV infections in Canada, 1987 to 2004. (*From* Bilsker D, Goldenberg L, Davison J. A roadmap to men's health: current status, research policy and practice. Vancouver, British Colimbia, Canada: Centre for Applied Research in Mental Health and Addiction and The Men's Health Initiative of BC; 2010; with permission.)

communities; the critically important areas of research to be explored; the male-specific or dominant health issues; and the diverse communities in which men of different ethnicities, races, and socioeconomic situations live, work, and play. The author thinks that the success of a provincial and national men's health strategy depends on the ability to

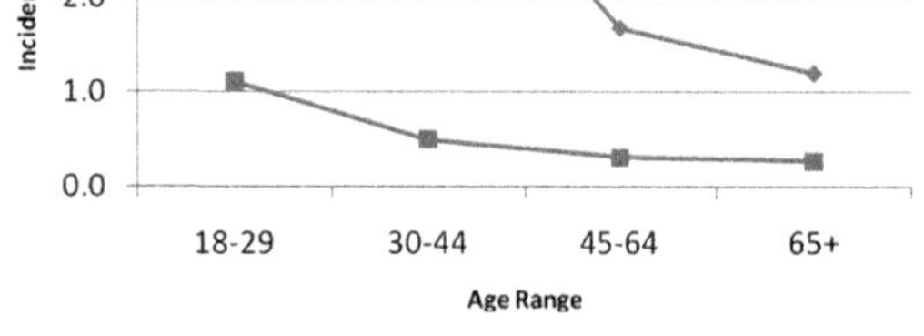

connect these dots, establishing a male-friendly, health-and-wellness oriented society as outlined in The Roadmap. In British Columbia, the critical connections are

The connection between foci of excellence Although there is expertise in different areas of male health, there is little in the way of collaboration, interconnectivity, and coordination. By forming a network in which experts in diverse fields and communities can communicate, discuss shared standards of care, share research opportunities, partner in grant applications, and interrelate electronically, the whole will far exceed the sum of the individual parts.

The connection between education, self-risk assessment, prevention, early diagnosis, and future health outcomes Many illnesses have risk factors and early signs and symptoms that are ignored or not recognized because of a lack of awareness. By helping men understand their individual, unique risks and vulnerabilities, they will have the option of modifying their behavior and attendance in health care systems to prevent future problems and achieve better outcomes in managing their illnesses.

The connection between different male health issues Over the past decade, it has become apparent that there are many linkages between

Fig. 11. Age and gender-specific incidence rates for alcohol abuse/dependence. (*From* Bilsker D, Goldenberg L, Davison J. A Roadmap to men's health: current status, research policy and practice. Vancouver, British Colimbia, Canada: Centre for Applied Research in Mental Health and Addiction and The Men's Health Initiative of BC; 2010; with permission.)

behavior, lifestyle, diet, activity, environment, workplace, employment opportunities, availability of social services, and the various illnesses that impact men across all age groups. As researchers, educators, health care administrators, and politicians plan the health care policies of the future, a male lens must be applied to help bring these linkages into focus.

The connection between regions: geographic and societal Although all men share a Y chromosome, the differences across the diverse cultures and societies in British Columbia are significant. The men of various socioeconomic status, races, ethnicities, and geographies should be connected through a common policy. These dots are diverse and unique, but the system needs to be adaptable to communicate with each in their own way and address unique concerns and needs.

The connection between male health care sectors The biopsychosocial issues that are male specific or dominant have different features and requirements when they are addressed in the greater community, in the acute care institutions, and in chronic care facilities. Standards of care and best practices need to be disseminated (developed where not available) within the context of our health care system to connect men's health issues across these sectors.

The connection between male health and wellbeing of other groups The approach to gender-specific community health is not an either-or question. Men's health policies, and ultimately improved health outcomes, must be connected as an equal partner to women's, children's, and minority health. Failure to address the health needs of any of these groups impairs the ability to fully serve the others.

MHIBC GOAL, MISSION, AND PRIORITIES

"Good design begins with honesty, asks tough questions, comes from collaboration and from trusting your intuition."
—Freeman Thomas, American automobile and industrial designer (http://quotesondesign. com/freeman-thomas/).

Goal

The MHIBC will help British Columbia's men improve their health and decrease their risk of disease, benefiting not only themselves but also the women and children in the families and communities that surround them.

Mission and Priorities

1. Reduce premature mortality rates among men by better understanding men's attitudes to health, investing in male-sensitive and culturally appropriate approaches to health care provisions, developing practical health promotion materials, reaching out to men to enable self-risk assessment, encouraging employer-based delivery of health checks and programs (well days), monitoring workplace hazards, initiating health care education early on in life for boys and young men in schools and diverse communities, and developing modern communication methodology to meet these goals.
2. Provide a multifaceted resource for health care practitioners across the Province of British Columbia through messaging, which is prioritized by professionals, independent of industry or media biases.
3. Create and coordinate a thriving men's health research environment, including a database of the health status and habits of men for public policy development.
4. Reduce the burden on our health care system by avoiding or delaying preventable illnesses and deaths in men through an extensive outreach communications and educational program and by developing cost-effective, community-based, male-friendly models for delivering services.
5. Develop a model of the multidisciplinary team approach to providing diagnosis, treatment, support, and leadership for the variety of physical, behavioral, psychological, sexual, reproductive, and social challenges of boys and men across the cultural and socioeconomic spectrum. This model would catalyze research and progress in a collaborative and practical setting, provide a site for the subspecialty development of best practices for disease prevention and management, and emphasize the role of the primary care physician as a care cocoordinator and health advocate.
6. Advocate for the development of coordinated provincial/national health and social public health policies for effective prevention and treatment programs based on evidence, standards of care, and best practices.
7. Fundraise and seek sponsorship for the development and sustainability of the required infrastructure and manpower, including academic chairs, to make the strategy a reality independent of volunteerism and free of industry influence wherever possible.

MHIBC EDUCATIONAL GOALS AND COMMUNITY OUTREACH

Many men, particularly in younger age groups, are unaware of their health-related risk factors and the impact of lifestyle and behavior on their health expectancy. Because so many boys and young men are less than anxious to read or be lectured about these issues, the MHIBC is aiming to reach them through social media–based communication programs, Internet-based interactive educational videos, digital media programs, and fun high school educational events. Messages may be delivered to middle-aged and older men via opportunistic outreach in the context of leisure activities such as has been done successfully through health clinics operating in barber shops or screening activities associated with sports events (hockey, soccer, and football in British Columbia).[33,34]

Working men will be accessed during working hours by partnering with major corporations, law firms, accounting firms, government agencies, and so forth. Male-specific health information will be disseminated through telephone-based centers, similar to the successful Men's Line Australia,[35] by communicating the information in a manner that is suitable to men's own priorities and perceived health needs. A speaker's bureau, community-based evening lecture series, dedicated medical journal publications, and Continuing Health Education (CHE) events for medical and nursing professionals are under development.

In all of these educational and outreach programs, we have to remain cognizant of the diverse sociocultural makeup of our communities in British Columbia. Gender roles tend to be even more pronounced in some ethnic minorities than they are among Canadian-born men. Public awareness programs to address alcohol abuse, spousal abuse, gang violence, unregulated natural and herbal remedies, and so forth, may be enhanced through an approach aimed at men of specific ethnic and cultural backgrounds. Lastly, tremendous opportunities for lifestyle-specific research, educational, and treatment programs exist in the gay men's communities of Vancouver.

MHIBC Research Goals

A recent analysis of funded health research in the United States and Canada found a substantial skew toward funding research on women's health. In Canada, between 2000 and 2005, men's health research received less than half the funding allocated to women's health by the Canadian Institute for Health Care Research and the Institute for Gender Health: 21% for men's health versus 52% for women's health research.[8] One of the reasons for this discordance may be historic in that differing academic perspectives generate men's health research that is confined to disciplinary silos. This point means that research relating to male health may even be taking place in several research programs at the same institution, preventing an integrated empirical understanding of men's health from emerging. Researchers from the biologic realm tend to conflate gender with biologic sex in relation to anatomic and physiologic aspects of male-specific or sex-differentiated health concerns, whereas social (qualitative) scientists tend to ignore the physicality of sex in preference to gender as a set of cultural and social constructs. Treadwell[36] stated: "To consider masculinity as dependent on innate biologic factors is to misunderstand the basis of genetics. But to consider masculinity as a purely social construct with no physiologic basis is scientifically dangerous." Recent science is now beginning to identify biologic manifestations of the impact of environmental, dietary, psychological, social, economic, and cultural circumstance, possibly through interesting epigenomic phenomena.

At the MHIBC, the author and colleagues are attempting to synthesize a broad range of disciplinary ideas into a meaningful framework that can easily translate into research team grants and highly valuable research productivity. The author's Roadmap has identified the need to (1) evaluate population-level initiatives to modify cardiovascular risk factors in men; (2) study male *suicide*, men's pathways to suicide, and population-level interventions to reduce its incidence; (3) investigate male *mortality from motor vehicle accidents*, emphasizing population-level interventions with younger male drivers regarding risk taking; and (4) compare treatment outcomes for male-specific conditions like prostate cancer and erectile dysfunction. The ultimate goal of the author's research programs is to bring disciplines together to achieve the research goals of translating findings into practice and policy contexts.

MHIBC Advocacy Goals

Men's health has climbed to a higher priority of decision makers and the public through the efforts of nonprofit groups committed to improving the status of men's health. The most prominent of these is the Men's Health Forum (MHF), founded in the United Kingdom in 1994, with activities extending across Europe. MHF states as its central belief that: "Public policy should aim to tackle health inequalities and barriers to good health in relation to gender as well as other health determinants."[37]

Advocacy by groups like this in Europe and Australia has greatly enhanced the profile of men's health in health care planning. There has been little such activity in Canada. Canadian men may be reluctant to participate in advocacy regarding their health or lack awareness of men's health as a crucial issue. Over the past decade, only one noteworthy men's health issue has received substantial media attention: an initiative to secure government funding for prostate-specific antigen testing for prostate cancer risk.[38] A Health Canada Web site ostensibly oriented to men's health offers only *generic* health care information on issues seen as relevant to men's health concerns.[39] An ambitious review of men's health issues commissioned by the Québec government 5 years ago had little impact on governmental policy.[40]

The MHIBC thinks that building healthy public policy is a core component of its male health promotion work. The author agrees with Geary[2] and Marieskind[41] in that the maturation of women's health as a domain for research and practice will serve as a model for the development of men's health. This development will require practitioners, researchers, and policy makers with an interest in men's health (or gender more broadly) to work in partnership to address and prioritize population-level initiatives that (1) adopt a male gender–appropriate approach, (2) integrate forms of communication well suited to men's identities, and (3) deliver interventions in settings that maximize access to men.

The MHIBC will seek a national men's health policy that is built around 4 foundation principles: gender equity, a focus on prevention, a strong and emerging evidence base, and an action plan to address needs across the life course. A gender-equity approach recognizes the different challenges that face men and women in managing their health, including their different health requirements and the different barriers they face in access to services. A focus on prevention will address behavioral, environmental, dietary, and socioeconomic risk factors. Health policy should raise awareness of men's health issues across the spectrum of age, race, socioeconomic status, and geography. It must relate to diverse issues, such as young men and suicide, prostate disease, alcohol misuse, obesity, hypertension, and sexual health. Male health does indeed go well beyond the penis and the prostate!

In 1999, Health Canada developed a women's health strategy that resulted in a gender-based activity and a well-funded Women's Health Network. An increasingly strong and influential men's health movement, consisting of health professionals, academics, and politicians, will have to adopt a broad gender lens within their efforts to raise awareness of men's health and develop a comparable men's health network in Canada.

CONCLUDING REMARKS

"You see things; and you say 'Why?' But I dream things that never were; and I say 'Why not?'"
—George Bernard Shaw, "Back to Methuselah" (1921), part 1, act 1.

The author thinks that British Columbia can become a global leader in men's health. MHIBC was created as a large-scale umbrella initiative aimed at connecting the dots by identifying, coordinating, and consolidating the existing foci of excellence across the many domains of male health in our province, enabling widespread education, risk assessment, prevention, screening, and early diagnosis. Through public and population health research and extensive outreach communication programs, the MHIBC hopes to improve men's health and quality of life by educating men of all ages (as well as their partners and families) about their risks and vulnerabilities and disseminating standards of care and best practices to professionals in all sectors of the health care spectrum. Each of the top 5 causes of PYLL identified in The Roadmap, which account for the gender life expectancy gap, have modifiable risk factors to be researched and mediated by carefully designed, implemented, and evaluated upstream interventions.

Gender is a key determinant of health, and the experience of being a man in our society affects our health and how it is managed. In the past decade, we have recognized the need to make men's health a distinct and important issue, much like the women's health movement. However, the science of male health is still very much in its infancy. Many questions need to be asked and answered on issues affecting all the ages and stages of the male lifespan. Each identified source of excess male mortality should be seen not as an indication of men's inevitable health disadvantage but rather as an *opportunity* to improve men's health status and longevity. Only by understanding the contributors to men's reduced life expectancy can we develop ameliorative interventions.

The time is now to look at health care through a male lens as the women's health movement has done productively for more than 30 years. The MHIBC will operate within a framework that highlights the key biologic, social, and cultural determinants and that recognizes that not all male population groups have the same health outcomes. We will create a discussion about the wide-ranging needs of men's health with governments, businesses, and the general public to ensure that the planning and delivery of health services better meet the needs of men and, in time, the development of a gender-specific action plan that identifies practical approaches to optimize health outcomes in men and boys.

REFERENCES

1. Minino AM, Heron M, Murphy SL, et al. Deaths: final data for 2004. CDC National Center for Health Statistics Web Site. Updated 2004. Available at: http://www.cdc.gov/nchs/products/pubs/pubd/hestats/finaldeaths04/finaldeaths04.html. Accessed July 25, 2009.

2. Geary MS. An analysis of the women's health movement and its impact on the delivery of health care within the United States. Nurse Pract 1995;20:27–8, 30–145.

3. A women's health strategy for British Columbia: advancing the health of girls and women. B.C. Women's Hospital & Health Centre and British Columbia Centre of Excellence for Women's Health Web site. Available at: http://www.bccewh.bc.ca/publications-resources/documents/pwhs.pdf. Accessed September 10, 2009.

4. Courtenay W. A global perspective on the field of men's health: an editorial. Int J Mens Health 2002; 1:1–13.

5. Available at: http://www.health.gov.au/malehealthpolicy. Accessed September, 2009.

6. Available at: http://www.dohc.ie/publications/national_mens_health_policy.html. Accessed September, 2009.

7. Bilsker D, Goldenberg L, Davison J. A roadmap to men's health: current status, research policy and practice. Centre for Applied Research in Mental Health and Addiction and The Men's Health Initiative of BC; 2010. Available at: http://www.aboutmen.ca/application/www.aboutmen.ca/asset/upload/tiny_mce/page/link/A-Roadmap-to-Mens-Health-May-17-2010.pdf. Accessed January 10, 2010.

8. Baerlocher M, Verma S. Men's health research: under researched and under appreciated? Med Sci Monit 2008;14:SC5–6.

9. Case A, Paxson C. Sex differences in morbidity and mortality. Demography 2005;42:189–214.

10. Oksuzyan A, Juel K, Vaupel JW, et al. Men: good health and high mortality. Sex differences in health and aging. Aging Clin Exp Res 2008;20:91–102.

11. Courtenay W. Constructions of masculinity and their influence on men's well-being: a theory of gender and health. Soc Sci Med 2000;50:1385–401.

12. Verbrugge LM. Gender and health: an update on hypotheses and evidence. J Health Soc Behav 1985;26(3):156–82.

13. Sabo D, Gordon DF. Men's health and illness: gender, power and the body. Thousand Oaks (CA): Sage Publications; 1995.

14. Rutz W. Men's health on the European WHO agenda. J Mens Health Gend 2004;1:22–5.

15. British Columbia Ministry of Health Planning. Selected vital statistics and health status indicators. The BC Ministry of Health Planning, Annual Report; 2002. Available at: http://www.vs.gov.bc.ca/stats/annual/2002/tab23.html. Accessed July, 2009.

16. Definitions and data sources. Statistics Canada health indicators, 2001, # 3. Statistics Canada. Available at: http://www.statcan.gc.ca/pub/82-221-x/01201/4149362-eng.htm. Accessed May 26, 2009.

17. Doessel DP, Williams RFG, Whiteford H. Policy-appropriate measurement of suicide: headcount vs. potential years of life lost, Australia, 1907-2005. Arch Suicide Res 2009;13:87–99.

18. Lai D, Hardy RJ. Potential gains in life expectancy or years of life lost: impact of competing risks of death. Int J Epidemiol 1999;28:894–8.

19. Tracking heart disease and stroke in Canada. Public Health Agency of Canada Web site. Available at: http://www.phac-aspc.gc.ca/publicat/2009/cvd-avc/pdf/cvd-avs-2009-eng.pdf. Accessed August 27, 2009.

20. Shah A. The relationship between suicide rates and age: an analysis of multinational data from the World Health Organization. Int Psychogeriatr 2007;19: 1141–52.

21. Bertolote JM, Fleischmann A. A global perspective in the epidemiology of suicide. Suicidologi 2002;7: 6–8.

22. Hu G, Wilcox HD, Wissow L, et al. Midlife suicide: an increasing problem in US whites, 1999-2005. Am J Prev Med 2008;35:589–93.

23. Hawton K. Sex and suicide: gender differences in suicidal behavior. Br J Psychiatry 2000;177: 484–5.

24. Varnik A, Kolves K, van der Feltz-Cornelis CM, et al. Suicide methods in Europe: a gender-specific analysis of countries participating in the "European Alliance Against Depression". J Epidemiol Community Health 2008;62:545–51.

25. Turner C, McClure R. Age and gender differences in risk-taking behaviour as an explanation for high incidence of motor vehicle crashes as a driver in young males. Inj Control Saf Promot 2003;10: 123–30.

26. Jonah BA. Age differences in risky driving. Health Educ Res 1990;5(2):139–49.

27. Hogg RS, Strathdee SA, Craib KJ, et al. Modeling the impact of HIV disease on mortality in gay and bisexual men. Int J Epidemiol 1997;26:657–61.

28. Hogg RS, Heath KV, Yip B, et al. Improved survival among HIV-infected individuals following initiation of antiretroviral therapy. JAMA 1998;27:450–4.

29. Hogg RS, O'Shaughnessy MV, Gataric N, et al. Decline in deaths from AIDS due to new antiretrovirals. Lancet 1997;349:1294.

30. Hogg RS, Strathdee SA, Craib KJ, et al. Gay life expectancy revisited [letter]. Int J Epidemiol 2001; 30:1493–9.

31. Alcohol dependence: Wikipedia entry. Available at: http://en.wikipedia.org/wiki/Alcohol_dependence. Accessed September 24, 2009

32. Miller T, Hendrie D. Substance abuse prevention dollars and cents: a cost-benefit analysis. Rockville (MD): Center for Substance Abuse Prevention, Substance Abuse and Mental Health Services Administration, DHHS Pub; 2009. No. (SMA) 07–4298.

33. White AK. Men's health in the 21st century. Int J Mens Health 2006;5:1–17.

34. Denner B, Bowering D. Centre for advancement of men's health: MAN model of health promotion. J Mens Health Gend 2004;1(4):393–7.

35. Men's Line Australia: supporting men and their families. Available at: http://www.menslineaus.org.au/. Accessed June 18, 2009.

36. Treadwell P. Biologic influences on masculinity. In: Brod H, editor. The making of masculinities: the new men's studies. London: Routledge; 1992. p. 259.

37. Available at: http://www.menshealthforum.org.uk/userpage1.cfm?item_id=1087. Accessed June, 2009.

38. Psa: To test or not to test? CBC News; 2009. Available at: http://www.cbc.ca/health/story/2009/03/19/f-prostate-cancer.html. Accessed July 21, 2009.

39. Healthy Living, Health Canada. Available at: http://www.hc-sc.gc.ca/hl-vs/jfy-spv/men-hommes-eng.php. Accessed June, 2009.

40. Wilkins D, Savoye E. Men's health around the world: a review of policy and progress across 11 countries. Brussels (Belgium): European Men's Health Forum; 2009. Available at: http://www.emhf.org/resource_images/11countries.pdf. Accessed November 21, 2009.

41. Marieskind H. The women's health movement. Int J Health Serv 1975;5:217–23.

Sexual Function in Men with Metabolic Syndrome

Richard K. Lee, MD, MBA[a,*], Bilal Chughtai, MD[a], Alexis E. Te, MD[a], Steven A. Kaplan, MD[b]

KEYWORDS

- Metabolic syndrome X • Obesity • Sexual dysfunction
- Physiologic • Urinary bladder • Overactive
- Waist circumference

The global epidemic of obesity and diabetes has led to a striking increase in the number of people afflicted with the metabolic syndrome (MetS). The MetS, or Syndrome X, consists of a constellation of abnormalities, including central obesity, glucose intolerance, dyslipidemia, and hypertension (HTN). These comorbidities constitute major risk factors for atherosclerosis and subsequent cardiovascular disease. Although interest in the MetS initially arose because of its association with cardiovascular disease, subsequent data have emerged pointing to a clear relationship with male sexual dysfunction. This review attempts to synthesize the data linking MetS and its impact on male sexual function.

DEFINITIONS

Definitions for the MetS are heterogeneous, as multiple sets of diagnostic criteria were initially created to identify insulin-resistant subjects or to predict clinical events, such as cardiovascular disease.[1] At present, 5 separate definitions for MetS exist (**Table 1**): the World Health Organization (WHO) working definition (1999), the European Group for the Study of Insulin Resistance definition (1999),[2] the American Association of Clinical Endocrinologists position statement (2003),[3] the Adult Treatment Panel III (ATP III) guideline

(2005),[4] and the definition from the International Diabetes Federation Consensus Group (2005).[5] Each of these definitions share certain common elements, such as criteria relating to obesity, hyperglycemia, dyslipidemia, and hypertension, but the laboratory value thresholds and the number of positive criteria required for diagnosis differ according to definition.[6,7] The ATP III definition is the one most commonly used today as it incorporates key concepts of MetS, relies on frequently used laboratory studies, and is less restrictive than the other classifications.[8] For the purposes of this review, the ATP III criteria have also been found to be the best predictors of arteriogenic erectile dysfunction (ED) and male hypogonadism.[9]

EPIDEMIOLOGY

WHO global estimates for obesity in 2005 reported approximately 400 million obese adults, or 9.8% of the population.[10] In the United States, this prevalence is expected to increase 40% for men by 2020, with the greatest increase in the superobese, that is, body mass index (BMI; calculated as the weight in kilograms divided by height in meters squared, ie, kg/m^2) of 50 or greater.[11–13] Correspondingly, the prevalence of the MetS in the United States has risen to

Extrainstitutional funding: None.
Financial disclosures: The authors have nothing to disclose.
[a] James Buchanan Brady Foundation, Department of Urology, Weill Medical College of Cornell University, 525 East 68th Street, F9 West, New York, NY 10065, USA
[b] Department of Urology, Weill Cornell Medical College, New York Presbyterian Hospital, F9 - West, 525 East 68th Street, New York, NY 10065, USA
* Corresponding author.
E-mail address: ril9010@med.cornell.edu

Urol Clin N Am 39 (2012) 53–62
doi:10.1016/j.ucl.2011.09.008
0094-0143/12/$ – see front matter © 2012 Elsevier Inc. All rights reserved.

Table 1
Definitions for metabolic syndrome

World Health Organization criteria (1999)	Presence of one of the following: diabetes mellitus, impaired glucose tolerance, impaired fasting glucose or insulin resistance, AND at least 2 of the following: Central obesity: waist: hip ratio >0.90 (male); or body mass index (BMI) >30 kg/m^2 Hypertension: $\geq$140/90 mm Hg Dyslipidemia: triglycerides (TG) $\geq$1.7 mmol/L and high-density lipoprotein cholesterol (HDL-C) $\leq$0.9 mmol/L Microalbuminuria: urinary albumin excretion ratio $\geq$20 µg/min or albumin:creatinine ratio $\geq$30 mg/g
European Group for the Study of Insulin Resistance (1999)	Insulin resistance defined as the top 25% of the fasting insulin values among nondiabetic individuals AND at least 2 of the following: Central obesity: waist circumference $\geq$94 cm Hypertension: blood pressure $\geq$140/90 mm Hg or drug treatment Dyslipidemia: TG $\geq$2.0 mmol/L and/or HDL-C <1.0 mmol/L or treated for dyslipidemia Fasting plasma glucose $\geq$6.1 mmol/L
American Association of Clinical Endocrinologists Position Statement (2003)	Insulin resistance AND at least one of the following: Central obesity: BMI$\geq$25 kg/m^2 Hypertension: >130/85 mm Hg or drug treatment Dyslipidemia: TG $\geq$150 mg/dL and HDL-C <40 Hyperglycemia Features of insulin resistance: family history of diabetes mellitus type 2 (DM2), polycystic ovary syndrome, sedentary lifestyle, advancing age, and ethnic groups susceptible to DM2
US National Cholesterol Education Program Adult Treatment Panel III (2005)	At least 3 of the following: Central obesity: waist circumference: $\geq$40 in (102 cm) Hypertension: $\geq$130/85 mm Hg or drug treatment Dyslipidemia: TG $\geq$150 mg/dL (1.7 mmol/L) or drug treatment HDL-C <40 mg/dL (1.03 mmol/L) Fasting glucose: $\geq$100 mg/dL or drug treatment
International Diabetes Federation (2005)	Central obesity AND at least 2 of the following: Hypertension: $\geq$130/85 mm Hg or drug treatment TG $\geq$150 mg/dL or drug treatment HDL-C <40 mg/dL Elevated fasting glucose: $\geq$100 mg/dL

approximately 35% to 39% of the current adult population.[14] The pediatric population has startlingly reflected this trend as well, with a doubling of overweight children in the past 30 years; this obesity is also associated with MetS features such as HTN, type 2 diabetes mellitus (DM2), and insulin resistance.[15]

SEXUAL DYSFUNCTION

A major limitation of the literature surrounding the impact of the MetS on sexual dysfunction revolves around the relative paucity of randomized trials. For example, no level 1 data exist regarding the impact of surgical treatment for the MetS on sexual function. Most data have therefore been drawn from cross-sectional or longitudinal studies, where association but not causation has been observed. In addition, the multiple definitions of the MetS have led to a lack of uniformity in how the MetS is diagnosed in relation to patients with sexual dysfunction.[6,7,16]

This article addresses sexual dysfunction as related to the MetS by stratification into two main categories, ED versus male hypogonadism or androgen deficiency. Although data in the literature have yet to support a causal relationship, the elements underlying the MetS are closely related with those of male sexual dysfunction and, in fact, successful treatment of the latter may influence the natural history of the former. Pathophysiologic mechanisms are explored here, as well as potential therapeutic paradigms.

Erectile Dysfunction

Multiple cross-sectional studies have documented a concordance between the causes of ED and cardiovascular disease, that is, elements common to the MetS.[9,17–25] This concordance was first reported by Gunduz and colleagues[18] who reported a 100% prevalence of the MetS in all 38 study patients with ED. In a cross-sectional study of 2371 men, Heidler and colleagues[23] noted that presence of the MetS, DM2, elevated waist-to-hip ratio, and HTN correlated with ED severity as defined by International Index of Erectile Function (IIEF) score, particularly in men older than 50 years. Bal and colleagues[24] demonstrated in a group of 393 men that the risk of ED increased with the number of MetS components, specifically waist circumference (WC) (odds ratio [OR] = 1.94), increased WC plus abnormal high-density lipoprotein (HDL) or triglyceride (TG) level (OR = 2.97), and increased WC plus pathologic HDL and TG (OR = 3.38). Demir and colleagues[20] demonstrated in a group of 89 patients with the MetS that ED as measured by IIEF–erectile function domain scores was correlated with the number of metabolic risk factors. Those with elevated fasting blood glucose, WC, or HTN had poorer erectile function compared with patients with other metabolic risk factors. It is interesting that Kupelian and colleagues,[21] using data from the Massachusetts Male Aging Study, have also demonstrated that the presence of MetS is associated with increased ED risk (relative risk = 2.09) even in those with a BMI of less than 25.

Erectile Dysfunction: Mechanisms and Pathophysiology

The MetS may lead to ED through multiple mechanisms (**Table 2**). Hypogonadism, which may be caused by the MetS, can lead to secondary ED through altered testosterone (T):estrogen levels. Corona and colleagues,[26] for example, demonstrated that low T levels were associated with greater WC and prevalence of MetS in a series of 1647 men with sexual dysfunction; T levels were inversely related to the severity of ED and directly related to the magnitude of penile blood flow in the oldest quartile of patients. T may affect the ability to achieve erections by helping to stimulate the expression of nitric oxide (NO) synthase and thereby increase the availability of NO in cavernosal tissue.[27] Atherosclerotic disease stemming from the same disease processes underlying the

Table 2
Mechanisms for metabolic syndrome–related erectile dysfunction

Mechanism	Comment
Hypogonadism	Altered testosterone:estrogen levels leads to hypogonadotropic hypogonadism; lowered testosterone leads to decrease in NO synthesis
Atherosclerosis	Damage to penile vasculature and cavernosal tissue leads to erectile dysfunction
Endothelial dysfunction	Decreased NO synthesis inhibits vasodilation; increased free radical production leads to atherosclerotic damage
Hyperglycemia	Glycation damage to penile tissues with resulting decrease in elasticity
Urogenital sensory neuropathy	Alteration in neural signaling to penis
Medications (eg, β-blockers)	Iatrogenically induced erectile dysfunction

MetS may also lead to ED by affecting the vascular tissues of the penis. Indeed, ED could be seen as a marker for occult coronary artery disease in otherwise asymptomatic men. Blumentals and colleagues,[28] for example, studied 12,285 men from the Integrated Healthcare Information Services National Managed Care Benchmark Database, demonstrating that men with ED had an almost twofold risk for acute myocardial infarction, even after adjustment for age at ED diagnosis, smoking, obesity, and use of angiotensin-converting enzyme inhibitors, β-blockers, and statins. Atherosclerosis can also lead to structural damage within the penile tissues. For example, Nehra and colleagues[29] demonstrated induction of penile smooth muscle atrophy and fibrosis in rabbit models for hypercholesterolemia and atherosclerosis. Koca and colleagues[30] reported on the relationship of the MetS on veno-occlusive dysfunction associated with ED in a group of 163 men. The MetS can also lead to endothelial dysfunction, which has been implicated in vascular disorders. Hyperglycemia, for example, induces a series of cellular events that increase the production of reactive oxygen species such as superoxide anion that (1) inactivates NO to form peroxynitrite and (2) increases oxygen-derived free radicals through activation of protein kinase C and other cellular elements.[31,32] Endothelial dysfunction therefore leads to a decrease in vascular NO levels, with resulting impaired vasodilation; the increase in free radical concentration also leads to atherosclerotic damage.[8] NO has been implicated in inhibiting platelet and leukocyte adhesion to vascular walls as well as decreasing smooth muscle proliferation.[33] Hyperglycemia can also lead to glycation of penile cavernosal tissue, leading to an impairment of collagen turnover and, potentially, ED.[34] Proinflammatory states, such as those found with DM2, can also lead to endothelial dysfunction through upregulation of E-selectin and altered tumor necrosis factor (TNF)-α:interleukin (IL)-10 ratio.[35] On a clinical basis, Pohjantähti-Maaroos and colleagues[36] reported on a group of 70 men with the MetS, where ED was shown to be correlated with decreased large arterial elasticity, independently of traditional cardiovascular risk factors. Long-standing diabetic neuropathy may also lead to urogenital sensory neuropathy, as reported in a series of 159 men by Bemelmans and colleagues.[37] The use of β-blockers for hypertension can also contribute to ED.[38]

Male Hypogonadism/Androgen Deficiency

Male hypogonadism, or androgen deficiency, has been defined by some investigators as total T levels 2.5 standard deviations below the mean in young adults or less than 319 ng/dL (11 nmol/L), although clinical criteria are more ambiguous.[39] Symptoms of hypogonadism include sexual dysfunction, fatigue, depression, irritability, hot flushes, decreased bone density, anemia, decreased lean body mass, and increased body fat.[40,41] The MetS has been associated with low T levels, with a particular effect in aging males.[42,43] Growing evidence now points to several potential mechanisms (**Table 3**).[26,44,45]

The first mechanism through which MetS may influence male hypogonadism is via leptin, a protein synthesized by adipocytes that regulates energy intake and use through influence over the hypothalamus.[46–48] Serum leptin levels have been shown to be directly correlated to BMI.[46,48] In addition, Luukkaa and colleagues[49] demonstrated in a cross-sectional study of 269 Turkish men that serum leptin levels varied inversely with T levels even after adjustment for BMI and insulin levels; administration of T to a cohort of 10 young men suppressed leptin levels until cessation of drug. Similar results were reported by Isidori and colleagues[50] in a group of 28 obese men compared with age-matched controls. Increased levels of leptin released as a result of increased obesity

Table 3
Mechanisms for metabolic syndrome–related male hypogonadism

Mechanism	Comment
Increased leptin levels	Decreased Leydig cell production of testosterone
Inflammation	Increased interleukin-1β, interleukin-6, and tumor necrosis factor α, leading to inhibition of testosterone production
Increased aromatase activity	Increased conversion of testosterone to estradiol leading to negative feedback on hypothalamus and hypogonadotropic hypogonadism

associated with the MetS may therefore decrease T levels, likely through a functional leptin receptor isoform on Leydig cells.[51] From a treatment perspective, T replacement or supplementation may decrease leptin levels and, therefore, obesity.[46,49]

The MetS also causes a low-grade proinflammatory state, which may also lead to or exacerbate hypogonadism. The inflammatory state created by the MetS is associated with increased levels of cytokines, specifically IL-1β, IL-6, and TNF-α, which inhibit T production.[52] TNF-α inhibits steroidogenesis at the nuclear receptor level, whereas IL-1 inhibits cholesterol side chain cleavage by cytochrome P450 in Leydig cells.[53,54]

The MetS is also associated with increased central obesity, which results in an increase in aromatase activity, facilitating the conversion of T to estradiol (E_2). Patients with the MetS should therefore have lower T:E_2 levels compared with controls. This finding has been confirmed by groups such as Vermeulen and colleagues,[55] who have demonstrated that obese men (BMI >35) have significantly lower T and higher plasma E_2 levels compared with controls. These obese men were also found to have a lower mean diurnal luteinizing hormone (LH) (LH level, LH pulse amplitude, and sum of LH pulse amplitudes); indeed, the decrease in LH pulse amplitudes was directly associated with lower T levels. This situation results in a functional state of isolated hypogonadotropic hypogonadism, likely stemming from the negative feedback of estrogen on the hypothalamus.[56] From a therapeutic point of view, Zumoff and colleagues[57] have studied the use of the aromatase antagonist testolactone in 6 obese men

(BMI 38–73) with hypogonadotropic hypogonadism, demonstrating a decrease in E_2 levels (from 40 to 29 pg/mL) with a corresponding increase in both LH (from 14.4 to 19.3 mIU/mL) and mean T levels (from 290 to 403 ng/dL), supporting the suppressive role of estrogens in pituitary gonadotropin production in obese males. Overall, the altered $T:E_2$ levels in patients with MetS can also cause further excessive visceral adipose deposition, leading to additional elevated aromatase activity, creating a positive-feedback loop, termed the "hypogonadal-obesity cycle."[58] This process has been demonstrated in studies such as those by Kupelian and colleagues[59] where hypogonadism was associated with a higher risk of developing MetS over time, particularly in nonoverweight, middle-aged men.

Treatment

Nonsurgical

Medical, or nonsurgical treatment, for sexual dysfunction associated with the MetS can target (1) the sexual symptoms resulting from the MetS as well as (2) different components of the MetS, for example, central obesity, hypertension, and insulin resistance.

At present, no direct pharmacologic treatment for the MetS exists; rather, lifestyle modifications in the form of diet change and physical exercise represent the foundation of therapy. Lifestyle modifications have been shown to improve endothelial function, decrease inflammatory marker levels, and prevent diabetes.[60–62] Specifically, Esposito and colleagues[61] studied 55 obese men with ED randomized to weight loss via reduction of caloric intake and increase in physical activity in comparison with a control group of 55 men. In addition to reduction in BMI, men in the treatment group showed improvement erectile function as measured by IIEF score. These men also showed reductions in IL-6 and C-reactive protein (CRP) levels, markers of inflammation. Changes in BMI, physical activity, and CRP levels in this study were independently associated with improvement in erectile function. Esposito and colleagues[63] also showed in a randomized, single-blind trial of 180 patients that the use of the Mediterranean-style diet, which consists of foods containing higher levels of phytochemicals, antioxidants, α-linolenic acid, and fiber (ie, fruits, vegetables, nuts, whole grains, and olive oil), is effective in reducing the prevalence of the MetS and its associated cardiovascular risk. Follow-up studies further demonstrated that adherence to the diet resulted in improvements in erectile function after 2 years.[64] Smoking cessation can also reduce oxidative

damage from carbon monoxide and increases the ratio of HDL to low-density lipoprotein (LDL) cholesterol, reducing atherosclerotic disease.[65] General principles to treat the different components of the MetS also include control of hypertension, hyperlipidemia, and insulin resistance.[66] Antihypertensive therapy should reduce blood pressure as close as possible to 120/80 mm Hg or lower. Statins should be used to reduce cholesterol levels. Medications such as metformin and thiazolidinediones, which reduce insulin resistance, can help regulate glucose metabolism. Of interest, Kim and colleagues[67] demonstrated that metformin activates adenosine monophosphate–activated protein kinase, thereby increasing the expression of neuronal and endothelial NO synthase, thus restoring NO synthase expression in penile tissue in mice and thus implying a potential benefit in humans.

Treatment of specific elements of sexual dysfunction include phosphodiesterase (PDE)-5 inhibitor and T replacement therapy (TRT) to address ED, and with the latter, hypogonadism as well. Sildenafil represents the prototypical PDE-5 inhibitor.[68] The performance of sildenafil in specific patient groups was examined in a meta-analysis of 11 randomized, controlled trials by Carson and colleagues[69] in 2002. Improvements in erectile function were found in 59% of patients with type 1 diabetes and 63% of patients with DM2, regardless of age, race, severity of ED, or the presence of various comorbidities. These response rates to sildenafil, however, were inferior to those in patients without diabetes (83%). The 2 other current PDE-5 inhibitors are tadalafil and vardenafil. Brock and colleagues[70] demonstrated a similar response with tadalafil in patients with diabetes. In a study of 1112 men with mild to severe ED due to various causes, 58% of patients with diabetes achieved erections sufficient for intercourse, compared with 75% of men without diabetes. PDE-5 inhibitors are contraindicated in patients using nitrates, due to risk of orthostatic hypotension.[71] Vardenafil is also not recommended in patients taking type 1A or type 3 antiarrhythmics.[72]

TRT can alleviate hypogonadism and thereby also help treat ED, in addition to having ancillary side effects on aspects of the MetS. Kapoor and colleagues[73] reported on 24 hypogonadal men with diabetes in a double-blind, placebo-controlled trial treated with intramuscular T versus placebo every 2 weeks for a total of 3 months. Treatment with T resulted in improvement in hemoglobin A_{1c} (HbA$_{1c}$) ($-0.37\% \pm 0.17\%$, $P = .03$), fasting blood glucose (-1.58 ± 0.68 mmol/L, $P = .03$), in addition to homeostasis model assessment (HOMA) index and cholesterol

(-0.4 ± 0.17 mmol/L, $P = .03$) levels. Reductions in WC (-1.63 ± 0.71 cm, $P = .03$) and waist-to-hip ratio (-0.03 ± 0.01, $P = .01$) were also seen. Boyanov and colleagues[74] reported on 48 men with DM2 and mild androgen deficiency in an open-label study where half of the patients were given T undecanoate and the other half placebo. Treatment with T resulted in statistically significant reductions in body weight (2.66%), waist-to-hip ratio (-3.96%), and body fat (-5.65%), in addition to improvement in HbA_{1c} from 10.4% to 8.6%. These results were echoed by Saad and colleagues,[75] who found that administration of T undecanoate over a 12-month period improved WC, plasma cholesterol, LDL, and HDL, with no side effects. Similar results, namely, improvements in WC, percentage of body fat, and total as well as LDL cholesterol, were found by Permpongkosol and colleagues[76] with similar medication in a group of 161 men with symptomatic late-onset hypogonadism. The impact of TRT was summarized in a meta-analysis of 5 randomized controlled trials by various groups who demonstrated significant improvements in fasting plasma glucose, HOMA index, triglycerides, HDL cholesterol, and WC, although not total cholesterol, blood pressure, or BMI.[42,77–80] The use of T, however, has not been without its potential side effects. Basaria and colleagues,[81] for example, reported on the use of T supplementation to increase muscle mass and strength in 209 hypogonadal men (total serum T 100–350 ng/dL or free serum T <50 pg/mL) aged 65 years and older with limitations in mobility. In a population with a relatively high prevalence of cardiovascular disease (47%–53%), diabetes (24%–27%), hyperlipidemia (50%–63%), and obesity (45%–49%), patients treated with transdermal T demonstrated an elevated risk for cardiovascular and dermatologic events (hazard ratio = 5.8) although greater increases in leg-press and chest-press strength and stair-climbing ability while carrying a load were seen. Because the trial was small in size and limited to a highly selected population, caution should be taken in administering T therapy. Overall, the small number of studies demonstrating the impact of TRT on insulin resistance or other elements of the metabolic syndrome in addition to the potential for deleterious effects in certain populations has led multiple organizations to not recommend such treatment in patients with MetS or DM2 in the absence of hypogonadism.[82] An ancillary method of treating the hypogonadotropic hypogonadism seen with the MetS includes the use of the aromatase inhibitor letrozole. Loves and colleagues[56] reported on an open-label 6-month uncontrolled trial in which 12 severely obese patients (BMI >35 kg/m^2) with hypogonadotropic hypogonadism were treated with 2.5 mg of letrozole weekly for 6 months. Use of letrozole produced a sustained normalization of serum total T, although free T levels rose to supraphysiologic levels in 7 of 12 (58%) men.

Surgical

Bariatric surgery represents an effective method to treat morbid obesity, albeit in highly selected patients. Patients must be motivated and able to participate in treatment and long-term follow-up, with clear and realistic expectations for how their lives may change after surgery.[83] As per the American Society for Metabolic and Bariatric Surgery "Rationale for the Surgical Treatment of Morbid Obesity" statement, patients whose BMI exceeds 40 are potential candidates for surgery if they strongly desire substantial weight loss because their obesity severely impairs the quality of their lives. Bariatric surgery may be considered in less severely obese patients (BMI 35–40) with high-risk comorbidities such as life-threatening cardiopulmonary problems (eg, severe sleep apnea, Pickwickian syndrome, obesity related cardiomyopathy, or severe diabetes mellitus) or obesity-induced physical problems that are interfering with their lifestyle.

Several studies have demonstrated that surgically induced weight loss can benefit sexual function. Camps and colleagues reported on a group of 94 patients who had undergone bariatric surgery and who experienced improvements in body image, enjoyment of sexual intercourse, and quality of orgasm, echoing earlier reports by Hafner and colleagues and Gahtan and colleagues.[84–86] More recently, Dallal and colleagues[87] studied the use of gastric bypass surgery in 97 male patients with morbid obesity. Increasingly heavier patients reported greater sexual dysfunction as measured by the Brief Male Sexual Function Inventory (BMSFI), but the amount of weight loss after bariatric surgery was significantly correlated with the subsequent degree of improvement in sexual function. Patients experienced improvements in sexual drive, erectile function, ejaculatory function, problem assessment, and sexual satisfaction after surgery, with BMSFI scores approaching those of reference controls after an average 67% excess weight loss. The role of weight loss by bariatric surgery on sexuality, however, is also incompletely studied, and one study demonstrating a negative effect on sexual function has been reported. Di Frega and colleagues,[88] for example, reported on secondary nonobstructive azoospermia with complete spermatogenic arrest in 6 previously fertile male patients who had undergone Roux-en-Y gastric bypass. Although gastric bypass provided sustained weight loss of 60 to 80 kg postoperatively, the nonobstructive azoospermia observed in these patients is concerning. The investigators hypothesized that this was likely secondary to nutritional deficiencies resulting from the bypass.[89]

Surgery specific for ED can also be performed. The introduction of the intrapenile prosthesis (IPP) by Scott and colleagues[90] formed the advent of prosthetic surgery for ED. The malleable penile prosthesis consists of a semirigid device with a central core allowing for the penis to be bent down for dressing and bent upward for coitus.[91] The positionable penile prosthesis (Dura II; American Medical Systems Inc, Minnetonka, MN)) is a semirigid device with a series of articulating segments held together with a spring on each end. The two-piece inflatable penile prosthesis (Genesis; Coloplast Corporation, Minneapolis, MN, and Ambicor; American Medical Systems Inc.) consists of two cylinders connected to a small scrotal pump allowing for easier implantation, but with the disadvantage of increased mechanical failure. The 3-piece inflatable penile prosthesis (Titan; Coloplast Corporation, and AMS 700; American Medical Systems Inc) possesses paired corporeal cylinders, a scrotal pump, and an abdominal fluid reservoir to most closely replicate penile flaccidity and erection.

SUMMARY

The MetS has become one of the major public health challenges worldwide. Interest in the syndrome initially arose because of its association with cardiovascular disease and diabetes in the setting of a growing worldwide epidemic of obesity. However, data have now clearly demonstrated its secondary impact on male sexual function. Effective and comprehensive treatment of male sexual dysfunction must therefore take into consideration treatment of any underlying elements of the MetS. The MetS appears strongly related to ED as well as hypogonadism. Few randomized studies exist to guide treatment of sexual dysfunction related to MetS; rather, most studies have been observational in nature. Medical therapy has formed the mainstay of treatment, with the advent of surgical intervention as a more recent phenomenon.

ACKNOWLEDGMENTS

The authors would like to acknowledge the assistance of Ms Kristin Saunders in the preparation of this manuscript.

REFERENCES

1. Corona G, Mannucci E, Forti G, et al. Hypogonadism, ED, metabolic syndrome and obesity: a pathological link supporting cardiovascular diseases. Int J Androl 2009;32(6):587–98.
2. Balkau B, Charles MA. Comment on the provisional report from the WHO consultation. European Group for the Study of Insulin Resistance (EGIR). Diabet Med 1999;16(5):442–3.
3. Einhorn D, Reaven GM, Cobin RH, et al. American College of Endocrinology position statement on the insulin resistance syndrome. Endocr Pract 2003; 9(3):237–52.
4. Executive summary of the third Report of the National Cholesterol Education Program (NCEP) expert panel on detection, evaluation, and treatment of high blood cholesterol in adults (adult treatment panel III). JAMA 2001;285(19):2486–97.
5. Adams RJ, Appleton S, Wilson DH, et al. Population comparison of two clinical approaches to the metabolic syndrome: implications of the new International Diabetes Federation consensus definition. Diabetes Care 2005;28(11):2777–9.
6. Chang ST, Chu CM, Pan KL, et al. Prevalence and cardiovascular disease risk differences for erectile dysfunction patients by three metabolic syndrome definitions. Int J Impot Res 2011; 23(2):87–93.
7. Guay A, Jacobson J. The relationship between testosterone levels, the metabolic syndrome (by two criteria), and insulin resistance in a population of men with organic erectile dysfunction. J Sex Med 2007;4(4 Pt 1):1046–55.
8. Huang PL. A comprehensive definition for metabolic syndrome. Dis Model Mech 2009;2(5–6):231–7.
9. Corona G, Mannucci E, Petrone L, et al. A comparison of NCEP-ATPIII and IDF metabolic syndrome definitions with relation to metabolic syndrome-associated sexual dysfunction. J Sex Med 2007;4(3):789–96.
10. WHO Consultation on Obesity Obesity: preventing and managing the global epidemic. Report of a WHO consultation. Wolrd Health Organ Tech Rep Ser 2000;894(1–12):1–253.
11. Flegal KM, Carroll MD, Ogden CL, et al. Prevalence and trends in obesity among US adults, 1999-2000. JAMA 2002;288(14):1723–7.
12. Sturm R. Increases in clinically severe obesity in the United States, 1986-2000. Arch Intern Med 2003; 163(18):2146–8.
13. Ruhm CJ. Current and future prevalence of obesity and severe obesity in the United States. Forum for Health Economics & Policy 2007;10(2)(Obesity):Article 6.
14. Golden SH, Robinson KA, Saldanha I, et al. Clinical review: Prevalence and incidence of endocrine and metabolic disorders in the United States: a

comprehensive review. J Clin Endocrinol Metab 2009;94(6):1853–78.

15. Deckelbaum RJ, Williams CL. Childhood obesity: the health issue. Obes Res 2001;9(Suppl 4):239S–43S.

16. Corona G, Mannucci E, Petrone L, et al. NCEP-ATPIII-defined metabolic syndrome, type 2 diabetes mellitus, and prevalence of hypogonadism in male patients with sexual dysfunction. J Sex Med 2007; 4(4 Pt 1):1038–45.

17. Corona G, Mannucci E, Schulman C, et al. Psychobiologic correlates of the metabolic syndrome and associated sexual dysfunction. Eur Urol 2006; 50(3):595–604 [discussion: 604].

18. Gunduz MI, Gumus BH, Sekuri C. Relationship between metabolic syndrome and erectile dysfunction. Asian J Androl 2004;6(4):355–8.

19. Esposito K, Giugliano F, Martedi E, et al. High proportions of erectile dysfunction in men with the metabolic syndrome. Diabetes Care 2005;28(5):1201–3.

20. Demir T, Demir O, Kefi A, et al. Prevalence of erectile dysfunction in patients with metabolic syndrome. Int J Urol 2006;13(4):385–8.

21. Kupelian V, Shabsigh R, Araujo AB, et al. Erectile dysfunction as a predictor of the metabolic syndrome in aging men: results from the Massachusetts Male Aging Study. J Urol 2006;176(1):222–6.

22. Grover SA, Lowensteyn I, Kaouache M, et al. The prevalence of erectile dysfunction in the primary care setting: importance of risk factors for diabetes and vascular disease. Arch Intern Med 2006; 166(2):213–9.

23. Heidler S, Temml C, Broessner C, et al. Is the metabolic syndrome an independent risk factor for erectile dysfunction? J Urol 2007;177(2):651–4.

24. Bal K, Oder M, Sahin AS, et al. Prevalence of metabolic syndrome and its association with erectile dysfunction among urologic patients: metabolic backgrounds of erectile dysfunction. Urology 2007; 69(2):356–60.

25. Yeh HC, Wang CJ, Lee YC, et al. Association among metabolic syndrome, testosterone level and severity of erectile dysfunction. Kaohsiung J Med Sci 2008; 24(5):240–7.

26. Corona G, Mannucci E, Ricca V, et al. The age-related decline of testosterone is associated with different specific symptoms and signs in patients with sexual dysfunction. Int J Androl 2009;32(6):720–8.

27. Reilly CM, Zamorano P, Stopper VS, et al. Androgenic regulation of NO availability in rat penile erection. J Androl 1997;18(2):110–5.

28. Blumentals WA, Gomez-Caminero A, Joo S, et al. Should erectile dysfunction be considered as a marker for acute myocardial infarction? Results from a retrospective cohort study. Int J Impot Res 2004;16(4):350–3.

29. Nehra A, Azadzoi KM, Moreland RB, et al. Cavernosal expandability is an erectile tissue mechanical property which predicts trabecular histology in an animal model of vasculogenic erectile dysfunction. J Urol 1998;159(6):2229–36.

30. Koca O, Caliskan S, Ozturk MI, et al. Vasculogenic erectile dysfunction and metabolic syndrome. J Sex Med 2010;7(12):3997–4002.

31. Beckman JA, Goldfine AB, Gordon MB, et al. Ascorbate restores endothelium-dependent vasodilation impaired by acute hyperglycemia in humans. Circulation 2001;103(12):1618–23.

32. Nishikawa T, Edelstein D, Du XL, et al. Normalizing mitochondrial superoxide production blocks three pathways of hyperglycaemic damage. Nature 2000;404(6779):787–90.

33. Creager MA, Luscher TF, Cosentino F, et al. Diabetes and vascular disease: pathophysiology, clinical consequences, and medical therapy: part I. Circulation 2003;108(12):1527–32.

34. Jiaan DB, Seftel AD, Fogarty J, et al. Age-related increase in an advanced glycation end product in penile tissue. World J Urol 1995;13(6):369–75.

35. Arana Rosainz MD, Ojeda MO, Acosta JR, et al. Imbalanced low-grade inflammation and endothelial activation in patients with type 2 diabetes mellitus and erectile dysfunction. J Sex Med 2011;8(7): 2017–30.

36. Pohjantähti-Maaroos H, Palomaki A. Comparison of metabolic syndrome subjects with and without erectile dysfunction - levels of circulating oxidised LDL and arterial elasticity. Int J Clin Pract 2011;65(3): 274–80.

37. Bemelmans BL, Meuleman EJ, Doesburg WH, et al. Erectile dysfunction in diabetic men: the neurological factor revisited. J Urol 1994;151(4):884–9.

38. Fonseca V, Jawa A. Endothelial and erectile dysfunction, diabetes mellitus, and the metabolic syndrome: common pathways and treatments? Am J Cardiol 2005;96(12B):13M–8M.

39. Vermeulen A. Androgen replacement therapy in the aging male—a critical evaluation. J Clin Endocrinol Metab 2001;86(6):2380–90.

40. Petak SM, Nankin HR, Spark RF, et al. American Association of Clinical Endocrinologists Medical Guidelines for clinical practice for the evaluation and treatment of hypogonadism in adult male patients—2002 update. Endocr Pract 2002;8(6): 440–56.

41. Kelleher S, Conway AJ, Handelsman DJ. Blood testosterone threshold for androgen deficiency symptoms. J Clin Endocrinol Metab 2004;89(8): 3813–7.

42. Corona G, Monami M, Rastrelli G, et al. Testosterone and metabolic syndrome: a meta-analysis study. J Sex Med 2011;8(1):272–83.

43. Kaplan SA, Meehan AG, Shah A. The age related decrease in testosterone is significantly exacerbated in obese men with the metabolic syndrome.

What are the implications for the relatively high incidence of erectile dysfunction observed in these men? J Urol 2006;176(4 Pt 1):1524–7 [discussion: 1527–8].

44. Kupelian V, Hayes FJ, Link CL, et al. Inverse association of testosterone and the metabolic syndrome in men is consistent across race and ethnic groups. J Clin Endocrinol Metab 2008;93(9):3403–10.

45. Goncharov NP, Katsya GV, Chagina NA, et al. Three definitions of metabolic syndrome applied to a sample of young obese men and their relation with plasma testosterone. Aging Male 2008;11(3):118–22.

46. Kapoor D, Clarke S, Stanworth R, et al. The effect of testosterone replacement therapy on adipocytokines and C-reactive protein in hypogonadal men with type 2 diabetes. Eur J Endocrinol 2007;156(5): 595–602.

47. Lee MJ, Fried SK. Integration of hormonal and nutrient signals that regulate leptin synthesis and secretion. Am J Physiol Endocrinol Metab 2009; 296(6):E1230–8.

48. McConway MG, Johnson D, Kelly A, et al. Differences in circulating concentrations of total, free and bound leptin relate to gender and body composition in adult humans. Ann Clin Biochem 2000; 37(Pt 5):717–23.

49. Luukkaa V, Pesonen U, Huhtaniemi I, et al. Inverse correlation between serum testosterone and leptin in men. J Clin Endocrinol Metab 1998;83(9):3243–6.

50. Isidori AM, Caprio M, Strollo F, et al. Leptin and androgens in male obesity: evidence for leptin contribution to reduced androgen levels. J Clin Endocrinol Metab 1999;84(10):3673–80.

51. Caprio M, Isidori AM, Carta AR, et al. Expression of functional leptin receptors in rodent Leydig cells. Endocrinology 1999;140(11):4939–47.

52. Kalyani RR, Dobs AS. Androgen deficiency, diabetes, and the metabolic syndrome in men. Curr Opin Endocrinol Diabetes Obes 2007;14(3):226–34.

53. Hong CY, Park JH, Ahn RS, et al. Molecular mechanism of suppression of testicular steroidogenesis by proinflammatory cytokine tumor necrosis factor alpha. Mol Cell Biol 2004;24(7):2593–604.

54. Lin T, Wang D, Stocco DM. Interleukin-1 inhibits Leydig cell steroidogenesis without affecting steroidogenic acute regulatory protein messenger ribonucleic acid or protein levels. J Endocrinol 1998;156(3):461–7.

55. Vermeulen A, Kaufman JM, Deslypere JP, et al. Attenuated luteinizing hormone (LH) pulse amplitude but normal LH pulse frequency, and its relation to plasma androgens in hypogonadism of obese men. J Clin Endocrinol Metab 1993;76(5):1140–6.

56. Loves S, Ruinemans-Koerts J, de Boer H. Letrozole once a week normalizes serum testosterone in obesity-related male hypogonadism. Eur J Endocrinol 2008;158(5):741–7.

57. Zumoff B, Miller LK, Strain GW. Reversal of the hypogonadotropic hypogonadism of obese men by administration of the aromatase inhibitor testolactone. Metabolism 2003;52(9):1126–8.

58. Cohen PG. Obesity in men: the hypogonadal-estrogen receptor relationship and its effect on glucose homeostasis. Med Hypotheses 2008;70(2):358–60.

59. Kupelian V, Page ST, Araujo AB, et al. Low sex hormone-binding globulin, total testosterone, and symptomatic androgen deficiency are associated with development of the metabolic syndrome in non-obese men. J Clin Endocrinol Metab 2006;91(3): 843–50.

60. Knowler WC, Barrett-Connor E, Fowler SE, et al. Reduction in the incidence of type 2 diabetes with lifestyle intervention or metformin. N Engl J Med 2002;346(6):393–403.

61. Esposito K, Giugliano F, Di Palo C, et al. Effect of lifestyle changes on erectile dysfunction in obese men: a randomized controlled trial. JAMA 2004;291(24): 2978–84.

62. Esposito K, Pontillo A, Di Palo C, et al. Effect of weight loss and lifestyle changes on vascular inflammatory markers in obese women: a randomized trial. JAMA 2003;289(14):1799–804.

63. Esposito K, Marfella R, Ciotola M, et al. Effect of a Mediterranean-style diet on endothelial dysfunction and markers of vascular inflammation in the metabolic syndrome: a randomized trial. JAMA 2004;292(12):1440–6.

64. Esposito K, Ciotola M, Giugliano F, et al. Mediterranean diet improves erectile function in subjects with the metabolic syndrome. Int J Impot Res 2006;18(4):405–10.

65. Goldstein MG, Niaura R. Methods to enhance smoking cessation after myocardial infarction. Med Clin North Am 2000;84(1):63–80, viii.

66. Borges R, Temido P, Sousa L, et al. Metabolic syndrome and sexual (dys)function. J Sex Med 2009;6(11):2958–75.

67. Kim YW, Park SY, Kim JY, et al. Metformin restores the penile expression of nitric oxide synthase in high-fat-fed obese rats. J Androl 2007;28(4):555–60.

68. Goldstein I, Lue TF, Padma-Nathan H, et al. Oral sildenafil in the treatment of erectile dysfunction. Sildenafil Study Group. N Engl J Med 1998;338(20): 1397–404.

69. Carson CC, Burnett AL, Levine LA, et al. The efficacy of sildenafil citrate (Viagra) in clinical populations: an update. Urology 2002;60(2 Suppl 2): 12–27.

70. Brock GB, McMahon CG, Chen KK, et al. Efficacy and safety of tadalafil for the treatment of erectile dysfunction: results of integrated analyses. J Urol 2002;168(4 Pt 1):1332–6.

71. Kloner RA. Pharmacology and drug interaction effects of the phosphodiesterase 5 inhibitors: focus

on alpha-blocker interactions. Am J Cardiol 2005; 96(12B):42M–6M.

72. Corona G, Razzoli E, Forti G, et al. The use of phosphodiesterase 5 inhibitors with concomitant medications. J Endocrinol Invest 2008;31(9):799–808.

73. Kapoor D, Goodwin E, Channer KS, et al. Testosterone replacement therapy improves insulin resistance, glycaemic control, visceral adiposity and hypercholesterolaemia in hypogonadal men with type 2 diabetes. Eur J Endocrinol 2006;154(6):899–906.

74. Boyanov MA, Boneva Z, Christov VG. Testosterone supplementation in men with type 2 diabetes, visceral obesity and partial androgen deficiency. Aging Male 2003;6(1):1–7.

75. Saad F, Gooren L, Haider A, et al. An exploratory study of the effects of 12 month administration of the novel long-acting testosterone undecanoate on measures of sexual function and the metabolic syndrome. Arch Androl 2007;53(6):353–7.

76. Permpongkosol S, Tantirangsee N, Ratana-olarn K. Treatment of 161 men with symptomatic late onset hypogonadism with long-acting parenteral testosterone undecanoate: effects on body composition, lipids, and psychosexual complaints. J Sex Med 2010;7(11):3765–74.

77. Heufelder AE, Saad F, Bunck MC, et al. Fifty-two-week treatment with diet and exercise plus transdermal testosterone reverses the metabolic syndrome and improves glycemic control in men with newly diagnosed type 2 diabetes and subnormal plasma testosterone. J Androl 2009;30(6):726–33.

78. La Vignera S, Calogero AE, D'Agata R, et al. Testosterone therapy improves the clinical response to conventional treatment for male patients with metabolic syndrome associated to late onset hypogonadism. Minerva Endocrinol 2008;33(3):159–67.

79. Aversa A, Bruzziches R, Francomano D, et al. Efficacy and safety of two different testosterone undecanoate formulations in hypogonadal men with metabolic syndrome. J Endocrinol Invest 2010; 33(11):776–83.

80. Tishova Y, Kalinchenko SY, Mskhalaya GJ, et al. The Moscow Study: a randomized, placebo-controlled, double-blind trial of parenteral testosterone undecanoate on the metabolic syndrome components and body composition. Endocr Abstr 2010;22:681.

81. Basaria S, Coviello AD, Travison TG, et al. Adverse events associated with testosterone administration. N Engl J Med 2010;363(2):109–22.

82. Wang C, Nieschlag E, Swerdloff R, et al. ISA, ISSAM, EAU, EAA and ASA recommendations: investigation, treatment and monitoring of late-onset hypogonadism in males. Int J Impot Res 2009;21(1):1–8.

83. American Society for Metabolic and Bariatric Surgery. Rationale for the surgical treatment of morbid obesity. Available at: http://www.asbs.org/Newsite07/patients/resources/asbs_rationale.htm. Accessed May 1, 2011.

84. Gahtan VV, Kurto HZ, Powers PS, et al. Changes in sexual patterns following vertical banded gastroplasty and weight loss. Obes Surg 1992;2(1):97–9.

85. Camps MA, Zervos E, Goode S, et al. Impact of bariatric surgery on body image perception and sexuality in morbidly obese patients and their partners. Obes Surg 1996;6(4):356–60.

86. Hafner RJ, Watts JM, Rogers J. Quality of life after gastric bypass for morbid obesity. Int J Obes 1991;15(8):555–60.

87. Dallal RM, Chernoff A, O'Leary MP, et al. Sexual dysfunction is common in the morbidly obese male and improves after gastric bypass surgery. J Am Coll Surg 2008;207(6):859–64.

88. di Frega AS, Dale B, Di Matteo L, et al. Secondary male factor infertility after Roux-en-Y gastric bypass for morbid obesity: case report. Hum Reprod 2005; 20(4):997–8.

89. Vazquez C, Morejon E, Munoz C, et al. Nutritional effect of bariatric surgery with Scopinaro operation. Analysis of 40 cases. Nutr Hosp 2003;18(4):189–93 [in Spanish].

90. Scott FB, Bradley WE, Timm GW. Management of erectile impotence. Use of implantable inflatable prosthesis. Urology 1973;2(1):80–2.

91. Montague D. Prosthetic surgery for erectile dysfunction. In: Wein A, editor, Campbell's urology, vol. 1. Philadelphia: Elsevier; 2011. p. 788–801.

Androgen Deficiency in Aging and Metabolically Challenged Men

Jeremy B. Shelton, MD[a],*, Jacob Rajfer, MD[b,c]

KEYWORDS

- Androgen deficiency • Late-onset hypogonadism
- Elderly • Metabolic syndrome

The life expectancy of both men and women has increased in the past century. As this population grows, androgen deficiency (AD) in aging men, or late-onset hypogonadism (LOH), is becoming an increasingly important issue that has engendered much debate among health care providers, including the government, insurers, and physicians. Greater insight into the pathophysiology of hypogonadism has fueled controversy about the benefits of testosterone (T) replacement in these men, with the hazards posed by cardiometabolic risk factors being of particular concern with the rising prevalence of such disorders among the elderly. This article reviews AD, the conditions associated with it, and its treatment. The complexities presented by maturing, metabolically challenged men are discussed.

PREVALENCE OF AD AMONG THE ELDERLY

The prevalence of AD among older men is thought to be high. Studies with inclusive (ie, strictly biochemical vs clinical) definitions of hypogonadism report high figures. In a longitudinal study of an aging prospective cohort, Harman and colleagues[1] cite the prevalence of low total serum T (<11.3 nM or 325 ng/dL) as 20% among men in their 60s and 50% among those more than 80

years of age. In another population-based study of community-dwelling men, Araujo and colleagues[2] found that, although almost one-quarter of those aged 30 to 79 years had low total T levels (<10.4 nM or 300 ng/dL), more than 18% of men aged 70 to 79 years had hypogonadism in conjunction with at least 1 specific symptom (low libido, erectile dysfunction [ED], osteoporosis/osteoporotic fracture) or at least 2 nonspecific symptoms of low T (sleep disturbance, depressed mood, lethargy, diminished physical performance). Even when using a more strict definition of LOH, in which at least 3 sexual symptoms were required in the presence of low total T levels, Wu and colleagues[3] showed that a significant proportion of older men had AD, with a prevalence of 3.2% in those aged 60 to 69 years and 5.1% in those aged 70 to 79 years. Given the variation in definitions and the need for uniformity, professional societies and consensus guidelines have recommended a standardization of LOH as total serum T less than the normal reference range of young, healthy men and clinical symptoms of AD.[4]

At current trends of population growth, it is estimated that the number of individuals aged 65 years and older in the United States will more than double between 2000 and 2030[5]; the proportion of older men with symptomatic and, thus,

The authors have nothing to disclose.

[a] Department of Urology, David Geffen School of Medicine at University of California, 10833 LeConte Avenue, Suite 66-124 CHS, Los Angeles, CA 90095-1738, USA

[b] Department of Urology, David Geffen School of Medicine at University of California, 10833 Le Conte Avenue, Suite 66-138 CHS, Los Angeles, CA 90095-1738, USA

[c] Division of Urology, Harbor-UCLA Medical Center, 1000 West Carson Street, Torrance, CA 90509, USA

* Corresponding author.

E-mail address: jshelton@mednet.ucla.edu

Urol Clin N Am 39 (2012) 63–75
doi:10.1016/j.ucl.2011.09.007
0094-0143/12/$ – see front matter © 2012 Elsevier Inc. All rights reserved.

potentially treatable disease is considerable and likely to grow.[2]

CONDITIONS ASSOCIATED WITH AD

The human and economic burden of aging-related decline in health is substantial. From sarcopenia and osteoporosis to depression and cognitive disorders, such debilitative disease processes are costly and widespread among the elderly.[6–9] Given the toll these often incapacitating afflictions take on the individual and on society, marked interest has developed in their prevention and treatment.

AD has been implicated in many of the conditions associated with aging in men. Changes in body composition, decreased bone density, depressed mood, and declines in cognition have been linked to low T, as have low libido and ED. Furthermore, maladies traditionally associated with cardiovascular and cerebrovascular disease, within a spectrum of disorders related to insulin resistance (variously known as the metabolic syndrome [MS], cardiometabolic syndrome, or syndrome X), have also been linked to AD. although not yet thoroughly elucidated, the relationship between AD and these risk factors for significant morbidity and mortality among the elderly presents both an intriguing opportunity for prevention and/or treatment of a wide variety of ailments as well as a cause for caution when considering T replacement for the androgen-deficient older man.

BODY COMPOSITION AND SARCOPENIA

Decreasing muscle mass and strength are associated with the aging process and are often accompanied by deterioration in physical function, mobility disability, and frailty, states that have been shown to predict quality of life, morbidity, and mortality.[10–13] In aging men, a concomitant decrease in T is observed,[1,14,15] and lower T levels have been associated with decreased muscle mass in epidemiologic studies.[16] This has led to the postulation that T plays a role in the development of sarcopenia, or loss of protein mass and function. Despite the known correlation between increased muscle mass and strength,[14] whether the effects of T are direct or indirect is not certain, which may explain disparate findings in the literature regarding the hypothetical downstream effects of sarcopenia on physical performance.

Observational studies have shown that higher T levels are associated with increased lean mass and decreased fat mass.[16–18] Interventional studies randomizing older men to exogenous T

or placebo have also shown favorable changes in body composition with T,[19–24] as has a trial with simultaneous 5-α reductase inhibition.[25] However, results are mixed for strength and physical performance, although several studies found significantly increased muscle strength among older men who received exogenous T,[19,23,24] investigations by Snyder and colleagues,[22] Emmelot-Vonk and colleagues,[20] and Kenney and colleagues[21] showed no difference between the treatment and control groups in domains of strength or physical performance.

Likewise, several prospective cohort studies reveal conflicting results. In a longitudinal examination of 2 independent samples, 1 nationally representative and 1 selective, Schaap and colleagues[26] showed no significant association between total or free T levels and either 3-year decline in physical performance or 3-year decline in muscle strength among older men. Conversely, Krasnoff and colleagues[27] showed that higher free T levels among the Framingham Offspring were significantly correlated with better physical performance and faster walking speed, whereas an increase of free T 1 standard deviation more than the baseline was associated with lower odds of either development or progression of limited mobility. In light of findings in another prospective cohort that (1) T levels in elderly men were significantly associated with increased lean mass and decreased body fat; (2) such characteristics in body composition were significantly associated with strength and physical function; but (3) T levels and physical performance were only weakly correlated at best; Araujo and colleagues[28] suggested that the influence of sex hormones on physical function may be mediated indirectly through body composition, indicating that the relationships between T, body composition, and physical function are not necessarily linear.

BONE MINERAL DENSITY

Osteoporosis and bone fracture among the elderly pose a formidable hazard to individuals and potentially a large burden to public health. Hip fracture has been well established as an independent predictor of morbidity and mortality among the elderly,[29–34] with more than 85% occurring among individuals more than 65 years of age in the United States[33]; the associated costs of care in the United States are estimated to be substantial.[35] Cohort studies of major bone fractures, in general, show older men to be at risk,[36] including one that observed older men to be at particularly increased risk compared with women and younger men.[37] An epidemiologic study of osteoporotic fractures suggests that the residual lifetime risk of fracture in men older than 60 years is high, approaching that of developing prostate cancer.[38] The modulation of bone metabolism by sex hormones has offered a compelling theoretic option for the prevention of osteoporosis and bone fracture through androgen supplementation, particularly among older men with both low T and low bone mass density (BMD).

However, although observational studies have shown that low T levels among older men are associated with increased risk of fracture (hip hazard ratio 1.88, 95% confidence interval [CI] 1.24–2.82, nonvertebral 1.32, 95% CI 1.03–1.68),[38] with increased falls,[39] with bone resorption,[39] and bone turnover products,[40–42] no interventional studies to date have shown an effect of T on the incidence of fracture. Multiple small, randomized, controlled studies have shown an increase in BMD with exogenous T; using transdermal formulations, Snyder and colleagues[22,43] showed a significant increase in lumbar spine density among treated older men with low baseline T levels, and Kenny and colleagues[21,44] found significantly increased BMD at the femoral neck among those with a low baseline free T who received exogenous T. Likewise, Amory and colleagues[45] observed increased BMD at hip and in spine with either T or T and 5-α reductase inhibition compared with placebo. Although a meta-analysis suggested that only intramuscular T was associated with increased lumbar BMD,[46] this did not include recent double-blinded, randomized, placebo-controlled trials, one of oral T among healthy older men in which no change in BMD was noted,[20] and one of transdermal T in a frail cohort of older men that showed an increase in axial BMD.[21]

Because no investigations of T administration have examined fracture as an outcome, treatment of osteopenia or osteoporosis with T has not been recommended by consensus groups.[4,47] In hypogonadal men, guidelines suggest monitoring of BMD and T at 2-year intervals.[4] Nevertheless, low T may be considered another useful clinical indicator in the global assessment of potential fracture risk among older men.[38]

FRAILTY

No agreement exists on the definition of frailty, but it has been recognized broadly as a decline in multiple organ systems leading to functional loss, diminished physiologic reserve, and increased risk of morbidity and mortality. Frailty is generally acknowledged as common among the elderly, although not necessarily as an inexorable result of aging. When examining multiple parameters including strength, ambulation, fatigue, weight loss, and comorbidities, several prospective cohort studies have observed an association between lower T levels and frailty, in cross-sectional studies[48,49] and over time.[50] One study also reported significant correlation between sex hormone–binding globulin (SHBG) and frailty,[51] although another examination of a larger cohort did not.[48] Because frailty encompasses many different states and processes associated with both aging and AD, evidence may not yet have reached a level for treatment recommendations, but the relationship does provide further information on the emerging picture of the change from physiology to pathology in aging and hypogonadism.

MOOD AND COGNITION

Although depression and AD prevalence increase with aging, a direct and independent association between the two has never been proven. However, a close relationship has been intimated by both observational and interventional studies.[52] Among the epidemiologic studies, low total T has been associated with more depressive symptoms in men of the Health Aging and Body Composition cohort[53]; low free T has been correlated both with increased risk of depression when adjusting for comorbid disease[54] and with increased incident depressive symptoms[55] in large samples of aged, community-dwelling men; and bioavailable T has been found to be 17% lower among men with depression compared with the rest of the Rancho Bernardo cohort.[56]

Interventional studies have shown mixed results for exogenous T therapy and mood. Short courses of T (12 months or less) in small study samples have tended to reveal some effect on mood, although differences between treatment and placebo groups have not been significant.[43,57,58] One study of treatment with low T doses (200 mg every 3 weeks for 12 weeks) showed no change in mood, although the putative aim of this particular pilot was to determine safety (ie, no other psychosocial effects of treatment) for therapy for cognitive decline in hypogonadal older men.[59] Positive studies include longer courses of drug exposure (up to 42 months)[60] or higher doses of drug.[61,62] Although other factors such as degree of AD severity may affect the neurophysiology of disease and treatment and are difficult to identify,[63] a meta-analysis of randomized, placebo-controlled androgen treatment trials for depression has suggested that T therapy is significantly associated with improved depression scores in both old and young hypogonadal men.[64] This analysis did not include a recent randomized, placebo-controlled trial of intramuscular T in 184 men with hypogonadism and MS, in which 30 days of treatment showed significant improvement in depression scores using validated instruments.[65] On balance, experts in psychiatry and neuroendocrinology have recommended T treatment of depressive mood associated with hypogonadism only in the research setting.[63]

A link has also been established between cognitive function and T, although, again, causative direction is not clear and other mediators seem to be involved. Observational studies have linked low free T levels with poorer cognitive function,[66,67] poorer memory,[66] dementia,[68] and Alzheimer disease,[69,70] with genetic risk factors playing an interactive role with hypogonadal states in Alzheimer disease.[71,72] A longitudinal study of older men revealed that those who developed a clinical diagnosis of AD also developed lower T levels in the previous 5 to 10 years,[70] offering a potential prospect for treatment if AD precedes clinical manifestations of cognitive decline.

Again, treatment studies exhibit differing results. Among investigations of healthy, older men, some report improved spatial cognition and memory following therapy with T,[73-76] whereas others show minimal to no effect on cognition with T[20,57,77] or T with finasteride.[78] Few small studies have examined treatment of men with mild cognitive impairment and/or Alzheimer disease; although 2 show some benefit with T therapy in visuospatial cognition and overall cognitive ability,[79,80] another showed no significant difference between cases and controls.[81] Once more, disparate findings convey the probable interplay between multiple observed and unobserved factors that contribute to the complex pathophysiology governing AD and cognition, as well as divergent methods in the studies themselves, including differing treatment duration, differing cognitive domains tested, and differing subject characteristics.[72,82]

LIBIDO AND SEXUAL FUNCTION

For most urologists, the primary contact with hypogonadism is made through men presenting with low libido, ED, or the side effects of androgen deprivation therapy (ADT) as treatment of prostate cancer. Much evidence exists linking low libido, suboptimal or absent sexual function, and AD. Population-based and convenience samples have correlated lower T levels with decreased libido and sexual function.[83,84] As noted by Wu and colleagues,[3] symptoms of sexual dysfunction proved to be more sensitive indicators of LOH than other symptoms of hypogonadism, such as

declining physical performance, depression, and fatigue. In this study of 3369 men aged 40 to 79 years, self-reported health status on multiple domains was correlated with serum T levels; symptoms that best predicted low serum T (<11 nM or 317 ng/dL) included low libido, poor morning erection, and ED.

Multiple studies have shown that T supplementation improves sexual desire and enjoyment, both in the short term[24] and with long-term therapy.[60] Moreover, it seems that T supplementation can improve response to phosphodiesterase type 5 inhibition.[85,86] In one investigation of diabetic patients with ED, a trial of sildenafil citrate revealed lower total T in those who did not respond to treatment; 70% of these nonresponders were converted to responders with coadministration of oral T.[85] T as monotherapy for ED has been shown to be effective in young men for whom hypogonadism is the primary cause of ED, but it was not in those with LOH.[87] Among hypogonadal men with major depressive disorder, T did seem to improve sexual function in both treatment and placebo groups such that the difference between the two was not significant.[88] However, older hypogonadal men receiving T showed significantly improved libido in a retrospective analysis,[89] whereas sexual function along numerous parameters improved with T compared with placebo in randomized treatment trials.[61,65] Similarly, significantly improved sexual function in the domains of spontaneous erection, sexual desire, and sexual motivation were observed in those receiving higher doses of T in a graded treatment trial compared with the placebo group.[58]

Although it is tempting to consider T therapy for such a well-established association as AD and ED, multiple studies and commentaries have noted that ED may be the consequence not only of low sex steroid levels but also of cardiovascular and metabolic disease.[90-94] As evidence builds suggesting a closer relationship between them without, as yet, a clear-cut sense of causative direction, so does concern given the theoretic increased risk of morbidity and realized adverse events recently posed by exogenous T exposure among those with cardiometabolic risk factors.

MS

Variously known as cardiometabolic syndrome, syndrome X, and Reaven syndrome, MS is distinguished by a constellation of hemodynamic and metabolic abnormalities, including maladaptive responses such as the glycemic dysregulation associated with visceral obesity. Hypertension and dyslipidemia are among the disorders represented that also increase risk for cardiovascular disease. Although the respective magnitudes of that risk contributed by each in this clustering of factors is still uncertain,[95] the cluster itself has, and continues to, become better characterized since the 1988 American Diabetes Association Banting Lecture in which Reaven coined the term syndrome X.[96] The 2 most current and widely accepted definitions of MS have been put forth by the International Diabetes Federation and the US National Cholesterol Education Program, both of which require increased waist circumference, blood pressure, triglycerides, and fasting blood glucose as well as decreased high-density lipoprotein (HDL) to establish disease.

At present, the prevalence of cardiometabolic risk factors among the elderly is high and seems to be increasing. In a 6-year period, the proportion of obese (body mass index [BMI] ≥30) US adults aged 60 years and older increased to 31% by 2004.[97] In another study of this nationally representative sample, greater than 15% of Americans more than 60 years of age had diabetes mellitus (DM), a likely underestimate of true prevalence given the high suspected rate of undiagnosed disease[98]; examination of a Medicare cohort suggested an increase of 23% in DM incidence between 1994 and 2004, with an increase in prevalence of 62% in the same period.[99] In a population-based national sample of US adults, the prevalence of MS was found to be greater than 40% in persons aged 60 years or older,[100] with increasing prevalence over time.[101]

The correlation between low T and MS has become the focus of intense investigation. Although the relationship is complex and the directions of causation not clear, advances in understanding have offered insights that ultimately present the clinician with a more difficult challenge regarding management of AD in an elder population given current evidence. On a biochemical level, the leading hypothesis for the underlying mechanism is the induction of hypogonadism by visceral fat through endocrine and cell-signaling functions. Negative feedback on the pituitary is postulated via aromatization of T to estradiol and production of the proinflammatory cytokines tumor necrosis factor a (TNF-a), interleukin (IL)-1, IL-6, and C-reactive protein (CRP).[94,95,102] Furthermore, leptin (a protein hormone produced by fat) seems to interfere with luteinizing hormone stimulation of androgen production.[103] Increased insulin likewise has been implicated in decreased testicular steroidogenesis.[95,104–106]

In vivo, 3 areas of research support a connection between T and MS: studies correlating low T with any or all of the cardiometabolic cluster risk factors; studies showing a link between ADT and MS; and studies showing that treatment with T may ameliorate many of the metabolic derangements associated with MS.[102]

Epidemiologic Studies

Multiple cross-sectional analyses have revealed that men with DM are significantly more likely to have low serum T levels. This association seems to be stronger in the elderly. In one study, the percentage of men with DM who had low T was nearly twofold higher than the percentage of men with DM who had normal T levels (64% vs 38%, respectively).[107] Another recent observational study of 2470 nondiabetic men more than 70 years of age found that progressively lower total T (<15 nM or 432 ng/dL) was associated with progressively higher rates of insulin resistance, independent of BMI, HDL, triglycerides, and age.[108] This association was not present for SHBG. In a survey of 580 men with type 2 DM, 43% had low total serum T and 57% had reduced calculated free T.[109]

A meta-analysis from 2006 reported a 42% pooled reduction in risk of DM among men with normal total T (15.6–21.0 nM or 449.6–605.2 ng/dL); of the 20 prospective and cross-sectional studies included, all found a statistically significant correlation between low T and DM accounting for age, race, and BMI.[95,110] Several longitudinal studies focusing on middle-aged men have also shown that low T is predictive of DM,[111,112] whereas another has questioned the role of T either as a causative factor in the development of disease or as an early biomarker for disease. In the Australian Longitudinal Study of Ageing, Chen and colleagues[113] found that low T in men more than 80 years of age did not predict incident DM in the 8-year study period; however, the investigators did note that total T levels were lower in men with DM than in men without, leading them to conclude that DM may result in low T, but low T does not seem to induce DM.

In a review of 2 lipid treatment studies, Kaplan and Crawford[114] noted that aging men with obesity and MS had lower T than aging men with neither; moreover, an association was observed between low T and various components of MS, including high triglycerides, obesity, and high serum glucose. This finding corroborates observational studies showing that T levels negatively correlated with triglycerides, total cholesterol, and low-density lipoprotein (LDL) and positively correlated with HDL.[115,116] Such associations may have some intuitive bearing on findings of low T and advanced atherosclerotic processes.

Low T has been associated with coronary artery disease[117–120] and carotid disease[121] in a graded fashion, with increasing degree of atherosclerosis as T decreases among older men. Although large-scale studies have not shown a direct or significant association between low T and incident myocardial infarction (MI),[122,123] an association has been shown between low T and incident stroke.[124] In addition to results from prospective cohorts such as the Rotterdam Study, in which low T was significantly associated with aortic atherosclerosis in older, nonsmoking men independently of age, BMI, DM, cholesterol, and HDL, this association suggests a potential direct effect of T on cardiovascular status.[125] The accumulated evidence has prompted some to classify low T as a cardiac risk factor.[116,118]

ADT

From a slightly different perspective, men undergoing ADT for prostate cancer (ie, men with medically induced, near-complete hypogonadism) have offered further evidence supporting a close relationship between T, DM, cardiac disease, and MS. The known sequelae of ADT include insulin resistance and vascular disease,[126,127] with many studies showing an increased risk of ultimate outcomes such as DM, MI, and increased mortality.[128–131] D'Amico and colleagues[132] found that 6 months of ADT significantly decreased time to MI, whereas Keating and colleagues[133] revealed that gonadotropin-releasing hormone (GnRH) agonist therapy, but not orchiectomy, was associated with increased risk of coronary artery disease, incident MI, and sudden cardiac death in a population-based cohort of more than 70,000 Medicare beneficiaries; the latter results were also found in a prospective study of more than 37,000 male veterans.[134] These findings are promising, but do not clarify whether the side effects of ADT mediate the pathophysiology witnessed or whether reduced T itself is responsible in this particular group of patients. Nevertheless, as Traish and colleagues[125] point out, it does seem that the reduction in T as seen with ADT is enough to initiate, promote, or initiate and promote this adverse progression of events.

In light of the current evidence, a recent consensus of the American Heart Association, the American Cancer Society, and the American Urological Association (endorsed by the American Society for Radiation Oncology) acknowledged the possibility and gravity of the relationship between ADT and cardiovascular risk with a statement that calls for prospective clinical trials and recommends to today's clinician that, although "there is

no reason at present to believe that there is a role for specific cardiac testing or coronary intervention in patients with cardiovascular disease before initiation of ADT,... prudence and good medical care dictate that patients with cardiac disease receive appropriate secondary preventive measures as recommended by the American Heart Association and other expert organizations, including, when appropriate, lipid-lowering therapy, antihypertensive therapy, glucose-lowering therapy, and antiplatelet therapy."[135]

Treatment Trials

Although treatment of AD, as measured by use of T replacement therapy (TRT), has increased in the last decade, estimates of the proportion of hypogonadal men receiving treatment are still low, at roughly 10% of eligible patients.[136–138] However, trials of AD treatment have proffered perhaps the most intriguing evidence for not only the relationship between AD and MS but the treatment of MS in the treatment of AD. Intramuscular T replacement in a small cohort of hypogonadal men with DM resulted in improved glycemic control and decreased insulin resistance compared with placebo.[139] Another small, single-blinded randomized trial of transdermal T with diet/exercise in hypogonadal men with MS and newly diagnosed DM saw 81.3% of men in the treatment arm no longer meeting criteria for MS, versus 31.3% in the diet/exercise arm, after 52 weeks.[140] A recent randomized, placebo-controlled, double-blind, phase III trial of 184 men suffering from both hypogonadism and MS showed T level normalization as well as significant decreases in BMI, waist circumference, and inflammatory markers (IL-1-b, TNF-a, and CRP) among those receiving 30 weeks of intramuscular T undecanoate compared with those receiving placebo.[105] These findings support those witnessed in a crossover trial of T in older hypogonadal men in which T replacement improved inflammatory cytokine profiles and decreased total serum cholesterol.[141] In a subsample of this study with ischemic heart disease, T replacement increased time to angina and ST segment depression in treadmill exercise testing,[142] corroborating results of an earlier trial studying men with stable angina and exogenous T administration.[143]

The early termination of a recent trial of T therapy in older, hypogonadal men has given pause to the otherwise alluring hope of T replacement in AD while simultaneously proving and complicating the relationship of T to cardiovascular risk and MS. During examination of the safety and efficacy of exogenous T in 209 older men with limited mobility, Basaria and colleagues[144] found a significantly increased incidence of adverse cardiac events in the treatment arm, necessitating the trial's cessation. A higher proportion of men in the treatment group carried cardiovascular risk factors at the outset, with significantly higher proportions of hyperlipidemia, antihypertensive use, and statin use. Nevertheless, multivariate analysis controlling for age, BMI, DM, hypertension, dyslipidemia, and HDL, and excluding the 104 men with self-reported cardiovascular, cerebrovascular, or peripheral vascular disease, still yielded increased odds for a cardiac event of 5.8 (95% CI 1.2–28.4) times that of the placebo group. Although this study does provide a cautionary tale on the safety of T replacement, particularly in metabolically compromised men with multiple cardiac risk factors, the investigators point out that the sample size was small, the number of events was small (28 cardiac-related events, of which 11 were considered adverse), that the study was not designed to examine cardiac outcomes per se, and that the types of cardiac events were diverse enough in nature to belie a single mechanism of causation (ie, T). Some have proposed that if the association is indeed causal, this may be because of the ability of T to increase motivation for, and tolerance of, exercise; in patients with multiple cardiac risk factors and poor functional status, these results may simply reveal the severity of cardiac disease and indicate that rapid increases in exercise tolerance may not be wise for this subgroup of patients. Many studies have been performed without significant complications among those treated. What this trial, among others, suggests is that the safety of and the patient selection for T replacement are still uncertain, and larger randomized trials are needed.[145,146]

With the overlap of androgen-deficient states, MS, and aging-related change, definitively attributing any of these disorders to AD and showing a benefit to T replacement thus continues to pose a challenge for clinicians and researchers. Despite incomplete comprehension of disease mechanism, a compelling claim and, arguably, pressing need for treatment remains, particularly with numerous studies showing increased mortality with T deficiency.[118,147–151]

MEASURING T

Measuring T has long been an inaccurate endeavor, adding to the challenges clinicians already face in terms of defining, diagnosing, and monitoring treatment of hypogonadism.[152,153] The normal ranges of T are not defined. The reference intervals for each assay differ. In addition, the range of T levels in patients varies by 3 orders of magnitude depending on age and presence of disease. Inaccuracy increases as T level decreases, rendering measurement of T in hypogonadal men and men on ADT particularly difficult.

In one study of reference ranges, Lazarou and colleagues[154] revealed that a 350% difference existed in the low end for total T (4.5–15.6 nM or 130–450 ng/dL) and a 325% difference existed in the high end (16.9–55.3 nM or 486–1593 ng/dL) across 25 US laboratories. Also showing the degree of variation seen between assays, Rosner and colleagues[153] cited the quality control program findings of the College of American Pathologists. Sending the same sample of blood from a hypogonadal man to 14 laboratories using 14 different assays, the total T measurement varied from 45 to 365 ng/dL (1.6–12.7 nM), with a mean value of 97.1 ng/dL and a standard deviation of 31.3 (3.4 nM and 1.1 nM, respectively). Even when looking at results from the single, most widely used instrument, which accounted for more than 30% of the laboratories, the total T measurements ranged from 65 to 130 ng/dL (2.3–4.5 nM).

There are 3 categories of measurement for androgen assays: direct immunoassay (radioimmunoassay, enzyme-linked immunosorbent assay, complement lysis inhibition assay); immunoassay after extracting T from serum by chromatography; and mass spectroscopy after extraction by chromatography. The cheapest methods are the least sensitive, specific, and accurate, but are the most widely used. Extracting T before measurement with immunoassay increases sensitivity and specificity, but remains imprecise. Mass spectroscopy is the most sensitive, specific, and reliable, but is the most expensive and the least widely used method of T measurement.[153]

Free T and bioavailable T are calculated based on measurements of serum total T (ie, T and SHBG). The performance of these tests is dependent on the performance of the total serum T measurement.

To address these issues, the Endocrine Society released a position statement on T measurement in 2007 that called for the use of the most accurate technology for standardization of assay validation.[153] In the interim, they recommend that providers know the exact assay used by their laboratory, know the assay's specific reference intervals, and, if possible, avoid the use of direct (ie, nonextraction) assays in hypogonadal men. They also call for a concerted effort to define the normal ranges for total and free T by age, gender, and disease state. Until this is done, they recommend the following: for adult men, the normal level of T should be greater than 320 ng/dL (11.1 nM); the definition of hypogonadism should be a T level less than 200 ng/dL (6.9 nM); the range of total T between 200 and 320 ng/dL (6.9–11.1 nM) should be considered equivocal; free T should be considered normal if it is greater than 6.5 ng/dL (0.23 nM); and bioavailable T should be considered normal if it is greater than 150 ng/dL (5.2 nM).

SUMMARY

AD is a prevalent condition whose associations with myriad age-related diseases responsible for significant morbidity and mortality among elderly men render it a disorder with tremendous potential individual and public health consequences in a rapidly aging population. Given the epidemiologic evidence of substantial overlap between low androgen states and states conferring a hazard of osteoporosis, cognitive decline, and metabolic dysfunction, among other unfavorable afflictions, the treatment of older men with LOH using T is intuitively attractive, if not promising. However, the disparate nature of findings among interventional trials suggests an incomplete picture of the complex interrelation between aging, AD, normal physiology, and pathophysiology, particularly given concerns for adverse events among those with cardiometabolic risk factors. To move beyond current guideline recommendations of highly selective therapy in symptomatic LOH on an individually considered basis, further in vitro and in vivo studies on proof of principle are merited, as are large, well-designed, and well-executed clinical trials to determine the safety and efficacy of exogenous hormone treatment. Until then, approaching androgen-challenged and metabolically challenged aging men will remain a challenge in itself.

REFERENCES

1. Harman SM, Metter EJ, Tobin JD, et al. Longitudinal effects of aging on serum total and free testosterone levels in healthy men. Baltimore Longitudinal Study of Aging. J Clin Endocrinol Metab 2001;86:724.
2. Araujo AB, Esche GR, Kupelian V, et al. Prevalence of symptomatic androgen deficiency in men. J Clin Endocrinol Metab 2007;92:4241.
3. Wu FC, Tajar A, Beynon JM, et al. Identification of late-onset hypogonadism in middle-aged and elderly men. N Engl J Med 2010;363:123.
4. Wang C, Nieschlag E, Swerdloff RS, et al. ISA, ISSAM, EAU, EAA and ASA recommendations: investigation, treatment and monitoring of late-onset hypogonadism in males. Aging Male 2009; 12:5.
5. Kinsella K, Velkoff V. US Census Bureau. An aging world: 2001. Washington, DC: US Government Printing Office; 2001.
6. Ernst RL, Hay JW. The US economic and social costs of Alzheimer's disease revisited. Am J Public Health 1994;84:1261.
7. Janssen I, Shepard DS, Katzmarzyk PT, et al. The healthcare costs of sarcopenia in the United States. J Am Geriatr Soc 2004;52:80.
8. Katon WJ, Lin E, Russo J, et al. Increased medical costs of a population-based sample of depressed elderly patients. Arch Gen Psychiatry 2003;60:897.
9. McCombs JS, Thiebaud P, McLaughlin-Miley C, et al. Compliance with drug therapies for the treatment and prevention of osteoporosis. Maturitas 2004;48:271.
10. Groessl EJ, Kaplan RM, Rejeski WJ, et al. Health-related quality of life in older adults at risk for disability. Am J Prev Med 2007;33:214.
11. Ling CH, Taekema D, de Craen AJ, et al. Handgrip strength and mortality in the oldest old population: the Leiden 85-plus study. CMAJ 2010;182:429.
12. Newman AB, Simonsick EM, Naydeck BL, et al. Association of long-distance corridor walk performance with mortality, cardiovascular disease, mobility limitation, and disability. JAMA 2006;295:2018.
13. Rolland Y, Czerwinski S, Abellan Van Kan G, et al. Sarcopenia: its assessment, etiology, pathogenesis, consequences and future perspectives. J Nutr Health Aging 2008;12:433.
14. Baumgartner RN. Body composition in healthy aging. Ann N Y Acad Sci 2000;904:437.
15. Purifoy FE, Koopmans LH, Mayes DM. Age differences in serum androgen levels in normal adult males. Hum Biol 1981;53:499.
16. Szulc P, Duboeuf F, Marchand F, et al. Hormonal and lifestyle determinants of appendicular skeletal muscle mass in men: the MINOS study. Am J Clin Nutr 2004;80:496.
17. Baumgartner RN, Waters DL, Gallagher D, et al. Predictors of skeletal muscle mass in elderly men and women. Mech Ageing Dev 1999;107:123.
18. Roy TA, Blackman MR, Harman SM, et al. Interrelationships of serum testosterone and free testosterone index with FFM and strength in aging men. Am J Physiol Endocrinol Metab 2002;283:E284.
19. Bhasin S, Woodhouse L, Casaburi R, et al. Older men are as responsive as young men to the anabolic effects of graded doses of testosterone on the skeletal muscle. J Clin Endocrinol Metab 2005;90:678.
20. Emmelot-Vonk MH, Verhaar HJ, Nakhai Pour HR, et al. Effect of testosterone supplementation on functional mobility, cognition, and other parameters in older men: a randomized controlled trial. JAMA 2008;299:39.

21. Kenny AM, Kleppinger A, Annis K, et al. Effects of transdermal testosterone on bone and muscle in older men with low bioavailable testosterone levels, low bone mass, and physical frailty. J Am Geriatr Soc 2010;58:1134.

22. Snyder PJ, Peachey H, Hannoush P, et al. Effect of testosterone treatment on bone mineral density in men over 65 years of age. J Clin Endocrinol Metab 1999;84:1966.

23. Srinivas-Shankar U, Roberts SA, Connolly MJ, et al. Effects of testosterone on muscle strength, physical function, body composition, and quality of life in intermediate-frail and frail elderly men: a randomized, double-blind, placebo-controlled study. J Clin Endocrinol Metab 2010;95:639.

24. Wang C, Swerdloff RS, Iranmanesh A, et al. Transdermal testosterone gel improves sexual function, mood, muscle strength, and body composition parameters in hypogonadal men. J Clin Endocrinol Metab 2000;85:2839.

25. Page ST, Amory JK, Bowman FD, et al. Exogenous testosterone (T) alone or with finasteride increases physical performance, grip strength, and lean body mass in older men with low serum T. J Clin Endocrinol Metab 2005;90:1502.

26. Schaap LA, Pluijm SM, Deeg DJ, et al. Low testosterone levels and decline in physical performance and muscle strength in older men: findings from two prospective cohort studies. Clin Endocrinol (Oxf) 2008;68:42.

27. Krasnoff JB, Basaria S, Pencina MJ, et al. Free testosterone levels are associated with mobility limitation and physical performance in community-dwelling men: the Framingham Offspring Study. J Clin Endocrinol Metab 2010;95:2790.

28. Araujo AB, Travison TG, Bhasin S, et al. Association between testosterone and estradiol and age-related decline in physical function in a diverse sample of men. J Am Geriatr Soc 2008;56:2000.

29. Aharonoff GB, Koval KJ, Skovron ML, et al. Hip fractures in the elderly: predictors of one year mortality. J Orthop Trauma 1997;11:162.

30. Keene GS, Parker MJ, Pryor GA. Mortality and morbidity after hip fractures. BMJ 1993;307:1248.

31. Lu-Yao GL, Baron JA, Barrett JA, et al. Treatment and survival among elderly Americans with hip fractures: a population-based study. Am J Public Health 1994;84:1287.

32. Magaziner J, Simonsick EM, Kashner TM, et al. Survival experience of aged hip fracture patients. Am J Public Health 1989;79:274.

33. US Congress, Office of Technology Assessment. Hip fracture outcomes in people age 50 and over—background paper (OTA-BPH-120). Washington, DC: US Government Printing Office; 1994.

34. White BL, Fisher WD, Laurin CA. Rate of mortality for elderly patients after fracture of the hip in the 1980's. J Bone Joint Surg Am 1987;69:1335.

35. Braithwaite RS, Col NF, Wong JB. Estimating hip fracture morbidity, mortality and costs. J Am Geriatr Soc 2003;51:364.

36. Jones G, Nguyen T, Sambrook PN, et al. Symptomatic fracture incidence in elderly men and women: the Dubbo Osteoporosis Epidemiology Study (DOES). Osteoporos Int 1994;4:277.

37. Center JR, Nguyen TV, Schneider D, et al. Mortality after all major types of osteoporotic fracture in men and women: an observational study. Lancet 1999;353:878.

38. Meier C, Nguyen TV, Handelsman DJ, et al. Endogenous sex hormones and incident fracture risk in older men: the Dubbo Osteoporosis Epidemiology Study. Arch Intern Med 2008;168:47.

39. Szulc P, Claustrat B, Marchand F, et al. Increased risk of falls and increased bone resorption in elderly men with partial androgen deficiency: the MINOS study. J Clin Endocrinol Metab 2003;88:5240.

40. Meng J, Ohlsson C, Laughlin GA, et al. Associations of estradiol and testosterone with serum phosphorus in older men: the Osteoporotic Fractures in Men study. Kidney Int 2010;78:415.

41. Szulc P, Garnero P, Marchand F, et al. Biochemical markers of bone formation reflect endosteal bone loss in elderly men–MINOS study. Bone 2005;36:13.

42. Tenover JS. Effects of testosterone supplementation in the aging male. J Clin Endocrinol Metab 1992;75:1092.

43. Sih R, Morley JE, Kaiser FE, et al. Testosterone replacement in older hypogonadal men: a 12-month randomized controlled trial. J Clin Endocrinol Metab 1997;82:1661.

44. Kenny AM, Prestwood KM, Gruman CA, et al. Effects of transdermal testosterone on bone and muscle in older men with low bioavailable testosterone levels. J Gerontol A Biol Sci Med Sci 2001;56:M266.

45. Amory JK, Watts NB, Easley KA, et al. Exogenous testosterone or testosterone with finasteride increases bone mineral density in older men with low serum testosterone. J Clin Endocrinol Metab 2004;89:503.

46. Tracz MJ, Sideras K, Bolona ER, et al. Testosterone use in men and its effects on bone health. A systematic review and meta-analysis of randomized placebo-controlled trials. J Clin Endocrinol Metab 2006;91:2011.

47. Bhasin S, Cunningham GR, Hayes FJ, et al. Testosterone therapy in men with androgen deficiency syndromes: an Endocrine Society clinical practice guideline. J Clin Endocrinol Metab 2010;95:2536.

48. Cawthon PM, Ensrud KE, Laughlin GA, et al. Sex hormones and frailty in older men: the Osteoporotic Fractures in Men (MrOS) study. J Clin Endocrinol Metab 2009;94:3806.

49. Wu IC, Lin XZ, Liu PF, et al. Low serum testosterone and frailty in older men and women. Maturitas 2010;67(4):348–52.

50. Hyde Z, Flicker L, Almeida OP, et al. Low free testosterone predicts frailty in older men: the health in men study. J Clin Endocrinol Metab 2010;95:3165.

51. Mohr BA, Bhasin S, Kupelian V, et al. Testosterone, sex hormone-binding globulin, and frailty in older men. J Am Geriatr Soc 2007;55:548.

52. Seidman SN, Walsh BT. Testosterone and depression in aging men. Am J Geriatr Psychiatry 1999;7:18.

53. Morsink LF, Vogelzangs N, Nicklas BJ, et al. Associations between sex steroid hormone levels and depressive symptoms in elderly men and women: results from the Health ABC study. Psychoneuroendocrinology 2007;32:874.

54. Almeida OP, Yeap BB, Hankey GJ, et al. Low free testosterone concentration as a potentially treatable cause of depressive symptoms in older men. Arch Gen Psychiatry 2008;65:283.

55. Joshi D, van Schoor NM, de Ronde W, et al. Low free testosterone levels are associated with prevalence and incidence of depressive symptoms in older men. Clin Endocrinol (Oxf) 2010;72:232.

56. Barrett-Connor E, Von Muhlen DG, Kritz-Silverstein D. Bioavailable testosterone and depressed mood in older men: the Rancho Bernardo Study. J Clin Endocrinol Metab 1999;84:573.

57. Haren MT, Wittert GA, Chapman IM, et al. Effect of oral testosterone undecanoate on visuospatial cognition, mood and quality of life in elderly men with low-normal gonadal status. Maturitas 2005;50:124.

58. Steidle C, Schwartz S, Jacoby K, et al. AA2500 testosterone gel normalizes androgen levels in aging males with improvements in body composition and sexual function. J Clin Endocrinol Metab 2003;88:2673.

59. Kenny AM, Fabregas G, Song C, et al. Effects of testosterone on behavior, depression, and cognitive function in older men with mild cognitive loss. J Gerontol A Biol Sci Med Sci 2004;59:75.

60. Wang C, Cunningham G, Dobs A, et al. Long-term testosterone gel (AndroGel) treatment maintains beneficial effects on sexual function and mood, lean and fat mass, and bone mineral density in hypogonadal men. J Clin Endocrinol Metab 2004;89:2085.

61. Cavallini G, Caracciolo S, Vitali G, et al. Carnitine versus androgen administration in the treatment of sexual dysfunction, depressed mood, and fatigue associated with male aging. Urology 2004;63:641.

62. Ly LP, Jimenez M, Zhuang TN, et al. A double-blind, placebo-controlled, randomized clinical trial of transdermal dihydrotestosterone gel on muscular strength, mobility, and quality of life in older men with partial androgen deficiency. J Clin Endocrinol Metab 2001;86:4078.

63. Ebinger M, Sievers C, Ivan D, et al. Is there a neuro-endocrinological rationale for testosterone as a therapeutic option in depression? J Psychopharmacol 2009;23:841.

64. Zarrouf FA, Artz S, Griffith J, et al. Testosterone and depression: systematic review and meta-analysis. J Psychiatr Pract 2009;15:289.

65. Giltay EJ, Tishova YA, Mskhalaya GJ, et al. Effects of testosterone supplementation on depressive symptoms and sexual dysfunction in hypogonadal men with the metabolic syndrome. J Sex Med 2010;7:2572.

66. Moffat SD, Zonderman AB, Metter EJ, et al. Longitudinal assessment of serum free testosterone concentration predicts memory performance and cognitive status in elderly men. J Clin Endocrinol Metab 2002;87:5001.

67. Yeap BB, Almeida OP, Hyde Z, et al. Higher serum free testosterone is associated with better cognitive function in older men, while total testosterone is not. The Health In Men Study. Clin Endocrinol (Oxf) 2008;68:404.

68. Hogervorst E, Combrinck M, Smith AD. Testosterone and gonadotropin levels in men with dementia. Neuro Endocrinol Lett 2003;24:203.

69. Hogervorst E, Bandelow S, Combrinck M, et al. Low free testosterone is an independent risk factor for Alzheimer's disease. Exp Gerontol 2004;39:1633.

70. Moffat SD, Zonderman AB, Metter EJ, et al. Free testosterone and risk for Alzheimer disease in older men. Neurology 2004;62:188.

71. Hogervorst E, Lehmann DJ, Warden DR, et al. Apolipoprotein E epsilon4 and testosterone interact in the risk of Alzheimer's disease in men. Int J Geriatr Psychiatry 2002;17:938.

72. Pike CJ, Carroll JC, Rosario ER, et al. Protective actions of sex steroid hormones in Alzheimer's disease. Front Neuroendocrinol 2009;30:239.

73. Cherrier MM, Asthana S, Plymate S, et al. Testosterone supplementation improves spatial and verbal memory in healthy older men. Neurology 2001;57:80.

74. Gray PB, Singh AB, Woodhouse LJ, et al. Dose-dependent effects of testosterone on sexual function, mood, and visuospatial cognition in older men. J Clin Endocrinol Metab 2005;90:3838.

75. Janowsky JS, Chavez B, Orwoll E. Sex steroids modify working memory. J Cogn Neurosci 2000;12:407.

76. Janowsky JS, Oviatt SK, Orwoll ES. Testosterone influences spatial cognition in older men. Behav Neurosci 1994;108:325.

77. Maki PM, Ernst M, London ED, et al. Intramuscular testosterone treatment in elderly men: evidence of memory decline and altered brain function. J Clin Endocrinol Metab 2007;92:4107.

78. Vaughan C, Goldstein FC, Tenover JL. Exogenous testosterone alone or with finasteride does not improve measurements of cognition in healthy older men with low serum testosterone. J Androl 2007;28:875.

79. Cherrier MM, Matsumoto AM, Amory JK, et al. Testosterone improves spatial memory in men with Alzheimer disease and mild cognitive impairment. Neurology 2005;64:2063.

80. Tan RS, Pu SJ. A pilot study on the effects of testosterone in hypogonadal aging male patients with Alzheimer's disease. Aging Male 2003;6:13.

81. Lu PH, Masterman DA, Mulnard R, et al. Effects of testosterone on cognition and mood in male patients with mild Alzheimer disease and healthy elderly men. Arch Neurol 2006;63:177.

82. Morley JE, Perry HM 3rd. Androgen treatment of male hypogonadism in older males. J Steroid Biochem Mol Biol 2003;85:367.

83. Travison TG, Morley JE, Araujo AB, et al. The relationship between libido and testosterone levels in aging men. J Clin Endocrinol Metab 2006;91:2509.

84. Zitzmann M, Faber S, Nieschlag E. Association of specific symptoms and metabolic risks with serum testosterone in older men. J Clin Endocrinol Metab 2006;91:4335.

85. Kalinchenko SY, Kozlov GI, Gontcharov NP, et al. Oral testosterone undecanoate reverses erectile dysfunction associated with diabetes mellitus in patients failing on sildenafil citrate therapy alone. Aging Male 2003;6:94.

86. Shabsigh R. Testosterone therapy in erectile dysfunction. Aging Male 2004;7:312.

87. Shabsigh R, Rajfer J, Aversa A, et al. The evolving role of testosterone in the treatment of erectile dysfunction. Int J Clin Pract 2006;60:1087.

88. Seidman SN, Roose SP. The sexual effects of testosterone replacement in depressed men: randomized, placebo-controlled clinical trial. J Sex Marital Ther 2006;32:267.

89. Hajjar RR, Kaiser FE, Morley JE. Outcomes of long-term testosterone replacement in older hypogonadal males: a retrospective analysis. J Clin Endocrinol Metab 1997;82:3793.

90. Diaz-Arjonilla M, Schwarcz M, Swerdloff RS, et al. Obesity, low testosterone levels and erectile dysfunction. Int J Impot Res 2009;21:89.

91. Esposito K, Giugliano F, Martedi E, et al. High proportions of erectile dysfunction in men with the metabolic syndrome. Diabetes Care 2005;28:1201.

92. Jackson G. Erectile dysfunction and vascular risk: let's get it right. Eur Urol 2006;50:660.

93. Kaplan SA, Meehan AG, Shah A. The age related decrease in testosterone is significantly exacerbated in obese men with the metabolic syndrome. What are the implications for the relatively high incidence of erectile dysfunction observed in these men? J Urol 2006;176:1524.

94. Traish AM, Guay A, Feeley R, et al. The dark side of testosterone deficiency: I. Metabolic syndrome and erectile dysfunction. J Androl 2009;30:10.

95. Guay AT. The emerging link between hypogonadism and metabolic syndrome. J Androl 2009;30:370.

96. Kalyani RR, Dobs AS. Androgen deficiency, diabetes, and the metabolic syndrome in men. Curr Opin Endocrinol Diabetes Obes 2007;14:226.

97. Ogden CL, Carroll MD, Curtin LR, et al. Prevalence of overweight and obesity in the United States, 1999-2004. JAMA 2006;295:1549.

98. Ford ES. Prevalence of the metabolic syndrome in US populations. Endocrinol Metab Clin North Am 2004;33:333.

99. Sloan FA, Bethel MA, Ruiz D Jr, et al. The growing burden of diabetes mellitus in the US elderly population. Arch Intern Med 2008;168:192.

100. Ford ES, Giles WH, Dietz WH. Prevalence of the metabolic syndrome among US adults: findings from the third National Health and Nutrition Examination Survey. JAMA 2002;287:356.

101. Ford ES, Giles WH, Mokdad AH. Increasing prevalence of the metabolic syndrome among U.S. adults. Diabetes Care 2004;27:2444.

102. Traish AM, Saad F, Guay A. The dark side of testosterone deficiency: II. Type 2 diabetes and insulin resistance. J Androl 2009;30:23.

103. Isidori AM, Caprio M, Strollo F, et al. Leptin and androgens in male obesity: evidence for leptin contribution to reduced androgen levels. J Clin Endocrinol Metab 1999;84:3673.

104. Carruthers M. The paradox dividing testosterone deficiency symptoms and androgen assays: a closer look at the cellular and molecular mechanisms of androgen action. J Sex Med 2008;5:998.

105. Kalinchenko SY, Tishova YA, Mskhalaya GJ, et al. Effects of testosterone supplementation on markers of the metabolic syndrome and inflammation in hypogonadal men with the metabolic syndrome: the double-blind placebo-controlled Moscow Study. Clin Endocrinol (Oxf) 2010;73(5):602–12.

106. Pitteloud N, Hardin M, Dwyer AA, et al. Increasing insulin resistance is associated with a decrease in Leydig cell testosterone secretion in men. J Clin Endocrinol Metab 2005;90:2636.

107. Tan RS, Pu SJ. Impact of obesity on hypogonadism in the andropause. Int J Androl 2002;25:195.

108. Yeap BB, Almeida OP, Hyde Z, et al. Healthier lifestyle predicts higher circulating testosterone in older men: the Health In Men Study. Clin Endocrinol (Oxf) 2009;70:455.

109. Grossmann M, Thomas MC, Panagiotopoulos S, et al. Low testosterone levels are common and associated with insulin resistance in men with diabetes. J Clin Endocrinol Metab 2008;93:1834.

110. Ding EL, Song Y, Malik VS, et al. Sex differences of endogenous sex hormones and risk of type 2 diabetes: a systematic review and meta-analysis. JAMA 2006;295:1288.

111. Kupelian V, Page ST, Araujo AB, et al. Low sex hormone-binding globulin, total testosterone, and symptomatic androgen deficiency are associated with development of the metabolic syndrome in nonobese men. J Clin Endocrinol Metab 2006; 91:843.

112. Laaksonen DE, Niskanen L, Punnonen K, et al. Testosterone and sex hormone-binding globulin predict the metabolic syndrome and diabetes in middle-aged men. Diabetes Care 2004;27:1036.

113. Chen RY, Wittert GA, Andrews GR. Relative androgen deficiency in relation to obesity and metabolic status in older men. Diabetes Obes Metab 2006;8:429.

114. Kaplan SA, Crawford ED. Relationship between testosterone levels, insulin sensitivity, and mitochondrial function in men. Diabetes Care 2006; 29:749 [author reply: 749].

115. Haffner SM, Mykkanen L, Valdez RA, et al. Relationship of sex hormones to lipids and lipoproteins in nondiabetic men. J Clin Endocrinol Metab 1993; 77:1610.

116. Maggio M, Basaria S. Welcoming low testosterone as a cardiovascular risk factor. Int J Impot Res 2009;21:261.

117. Jones RD, Malkin CJ, Channer KS, et al. Low levels of endogenous androgens increase the risk of atherosclerosis in elderly men: further supportive data. J Clin Endocrinol Metab 2003;88:1403.

118. Khaw KT, Dowsett M, Folkerd E, et al. Endogenous testosterone and mortality due to all causes, cardiovascular disease, and cancer in men: European prospective investigation into cancer in Norfolk (EPIC-Norfolk) Prospective Population Study. Circulation 2007;116:2694.

119. Phillips GB, Pinkernell BH, Jing TY. The association of hypotestosteronemia with coronary artery disease in men. Arterioscler Thromb 1994;14:701.

120. Rosano GM, Sheiban I, Massaro R, et al. Low testosterone levels are associated with coronary artery disease in male patients with angina. Int J Impot Res 2007;19:176.

121. Muller M, van den Beld AW, Bots ML, et al. Endogenous sex hormones and progression of carotid atherosclerosis in elderly men. Circulation 2004; 109:2074.

122. Militaru C, Donoiu I, Dracea O, et al. Serum testosterone and short-term mortality in men with acute myocardial infarction. Cardiol J 2010;17:249.

123. Vikan T, Schirmer H, Njolstad I, et al. Endogenous sex hormones and the prospective association with cardiovascular disease and mortality in men: the Tromso Study. Eur J Endocrinol 2009;161:435.

124. Yeap BB, Hyde Z, Almeida OP, et al. Lower testosterone levels predict incident stroke and transient ischemic attack in older men. J Clin Endocrinol Metab 2009;94:2353.

125. Traish AM, Saad F, Feeley RJ, et al. The dark side of testosterone deficiency: III. Cardiovascular disease. J Androl 2009;30:477.

126. Basaria S, Muller DC, Carducci MA, et al. Hyperglycemia and insulin resistance in men with prostate carcinoma who receive androgen-deprivation therapy. Cancer 2006;106:581.

127. Shahani S, Braga-Basaria M, Basaria S. Androgen deprivation therapy in prostate cancer and metabolic risk for atherosclerosis. J Clin Endocrinol Metab 2008;93:2042.

128. Hakimian P, Blute M Jr, Kashanian J, et al. Metabolic and cardiovascular effects of androgen deprivation therapy. BJU Int 2008;102:1509.

129. Platz EA. Low testosterone and risk of premature death in older men: analytical and preanalytical issues in measuring circulating testosterone. Clin Chem 2008;54:1110.

130. Saigal CS, Gore JL, Krupski TL, et al. Androgen deprivation therapy increases cardiovascular morbidity in men with prostate cancer. Cancer 2007;110:1493.

131. Tsai HK, D'Amico AV, Sadetsky N, et al. Androgen deprivation therapy for localized prostate cancer and the risk of cardiovascular mortality. J Natl Cancer Inst 2007;99:1516.

132. D'Amico AV, Denham JW, Crook J, et al. Influence of androgen suppression therapy for prostate cancer on the frequency and timing of fatal myocardial infarctions. J Clin Oncol 2007;25:2420.

133. Keating NL, O'Malley AJ, Smith MR. Diabetes and cardiovascular disease during androgen deprivation therapy for prostate cancer. J Clin Oncol 2006;24:4448.

134. Keating NL, O'Malley AJ, Freedland SJ, et al. Diabetes and cardiovascular disease during androgen deprivation therapy: observational study of veterans with prostate cancer. J Natl Cancer Inst 2010;102:39.

135. Levine GN, D'Amico AV, Berger P, et al. Androgen-deprivation therapy in prostate cancer and cardiovascular risk: a science advisory from the American Heart Association, American Cancer Society, and American Urological Association: endorsed by the American Society for Radiation Oncology. Circulation 2010;121:833.

136. Carruthers M. Time for international action on treating testosterone deficiency syndrome. Aging Male 2009;12:21.

137. Hall SA, Araujo AB, Esche GR, et al. Treatment of symptomatic androgen deficiency: results from the Boston Area Community Health Survey. Arch Intern Med 2008;168:1070.

138. Mulligan T, Frick MF, Zuraw QC, et al. Prevalence of hypogonadism in males aged at least 45 years: the HIM study. Int J Clin Pract 2006;60:762.

139. Kapoor D, Goodwin E, Channer KS, et al. Testosterone replacement therapy improves insulin resistance, glycaemic control, visceral adiposity and hypercholesterolaemia in hypogonadal men with type 2 diabetes. Eur J Endocrinol 2006;154:899.

140. Heufelder AE, Saad F, Bunck MC, et al. Fifty-two-week treatment with diet and exercise plus transdermal testosterone reverses the metabolic syndrome and improves glycemic control in men with newly diagnosed type 2 diabetes and subnormal plasma testosterone. J Androl 2009;30:726.

141. Malkin CJ, Pugh PJ, Jones RD, et al. The effect of testosterone replacement on endogenous inflammatory cytokines and lipid profiles in hypogonadal men. J Clin Endocrinol Metab 2004;89:3313.

142. Malkin CJ, Pugh PJ, Morris PD, et al. Testosterone replacement in hypogonadal men with angina improves ischaemic threshold and quality of life. Heart 2004;90:871.

143. English KM, Steeds RP, Jones TH, et al. Low-dose transdermal testosterone therapy improves angina threshold in men with chronic stable angina: a randomized, double-blind, placebo-controlled study. Circulation 2000;102:1906.

144. Basaria S, Coviello AD, Travison TG, et al. Adverse events associated with testosterone administration. N Engl J Med 2010;363:109.

145. Fernandez-Balsells MM, Murad MH, Lane M, et al. Clinical review 1: adverse effects of testosterone therapy in adult men: a systematic review and meta-analysis. J Clin Endocrinol Metab 2010;95: 2560.

146. Haddad RM, Kennedy CC, Caples SM, et al. Testosterone and cardiovascular risk in men: a systematic review and meta-analysis of randomized placebo-controlled trials. Mayo Clin Proc 2007;82:29.

147. Araujo AB, Kupelian V, Page ST, et al. Sex steroids and all-cause and cause-specific mortality in men. Arch Intern Med 2007;167:1252.

148. Laughlin GA, Barrett-Connor E, Bergstrom J. Low serum testosterone and mortality in older men. J Clin Endocrinol Metab 2008;93:68.

149. Laughlin GA, Goodell V, Barrett-Connor E. Extremes of endogenous testosterone are associated with increased risk of incident coronary events in older women. J Clin Endocrinol Metab 2010;95:740.

150. Maggio M, Lauretani F, Ceda GP, et al. Relationship between low levels of anabolic hormones and 6-year mortality in older men: the aging in the Chianti Area (InCHIANTI) study. Arch Intern Med 2007; 167:2249.

151. Shores MM, Matsumoto AM, Sloan KL, et al. Low serum testosterone and mortality in male veterans. Arch Intern Med 2006;166:1660.

152. Carruthers M, Trinick TR, Wheeler MJ. The validity of androgen assays. Aging Male 2007;10:165.

153. Rosner W, Auchus RJ, Azziz R, et al. Position statement: utility, limitations, and pitfalls in measuring testosterone: an Endocrine Society position statement. J Clin Endocrinol Metab 2007;92:405.

154. Lazarou S, Reyes-Vallejo L, Morgentaler A. Wide variability in laboratory reference values for serum testosterone. J Sex Med 2006;3:1085.

Influences of Neuroregulatory Factors on the Development of Lower Urinary Tract Symptoms/Benign Prostatic Hyperplasia and Erectile Dysfunction in Aging Men

Daniel J. Mazur, MD, Brian T. Helfand, MD, PhD,
Kevin T. McVary, MD*

KEYWORDS

- Aging • Neuroregulatory factors
- Lower urinary tract symptoms
- Benign prostatic hyperplasia • Erectile dysfunction
- Metabolic syndrome

As men age, there is an associated increase in the frequency of pathologic diseases affecting the genitourinary tract. Most notable among these changes are the rising prevalence of lower urinary tract symptoms (LUTS) secondary to benign prostatic hyperplasia (BPH) and erectile dysfunction (ED). The pathogenesis of these conditions seems to be multifactorial and includes age-related changes in the nervous system and neuroregulatory factors, such as nitric oxide (NO) and RhoA/Rho-kinase. Although some of these neuromodulatory effects are directly associated with the aging process, many are secondary to comorbid conditions related to aging, such as the metabolic syndrome (MSx), diabetes, and hypogonadism. The success of several widely used pharmacologic interventions reflect the importance of neuronal influences on urologic disease in aging men.

NORMAL INNERVATION OF THE BLADDER, PROSTATE, AND PENIS

The male lower urinary tract is innervated by both the somatic and the autonomic nervous systems (ANS). The autonomic component consists of pelvic parasympathetic and lumbar sympathetic nerves. In addition, the role of other neuroregulatory pathways, such as NO and RhoA/Rho-kinase, are

Disclosures: McVary is an investigator/consultant for NIDDK, Allergan, Eli Lilly, and a consultant for GSK and Watson; Helfand and Mazur have nothing to disclose.
Department of Urology, Northwestern University Feinberg School of Medicine, 303 East Chicago Avenue, Tarry 16-703, Chicago, IL 60611-3008, USA
* Corresponding author.
E-mail address: k-mcvary@northwestern.edu

Urol Clin N Am 39 (2012) 77–88
doi:10.1016/j.ucl.2011.09.005
0094-0143/12/$ – see front matter © 2012 Elsevier Inc. All rights reserved.

increasing being described in the lower urinary tract. These nerves serve important roles in the regulation of urine storage, micturition, erectile function, and ejaculation.

Bladder

Parasympathetic nerves help to control micturition through innervation of bladder detrusor muscles (**Fig. 1**). This interaction is mediated by acetylcholine (ACh) binding to detrusor muscarinic receptors. There are 5 subtypes of muscarinic receptors.[1] Although there is more expression of the M_2 subtype in the bladder, the M_3 subtype is the most important for initiating detrusor contractions.[2,3]

Muscarinic receptor binding leads to a cascade of signaling events that results in the activation of phospholipase C (PLC) and the hydrolysis of inositol 1,4,5-trisphosphate (IP_3). Subsequently, IP_3 causes an increase in intracellular calcium, which binds calmodulin (CaM) to activate myosin light chain kinase (MLCK). Phosphorylation of myosin regulatory light chain (MLC) by MLCK causes MLC to activate myosin ATPase and enhance muscle contractility. MLC is dephosphorylated by MLC phosphatase (MLCP), which results in muscle relaxation.[4] In addition, smooth muscle cell (SMC) contraction is also regulated through the RhoA/Rho-kinase pathway, also called the alternate pathway.[5] Activation of Rho-kinase occurs through

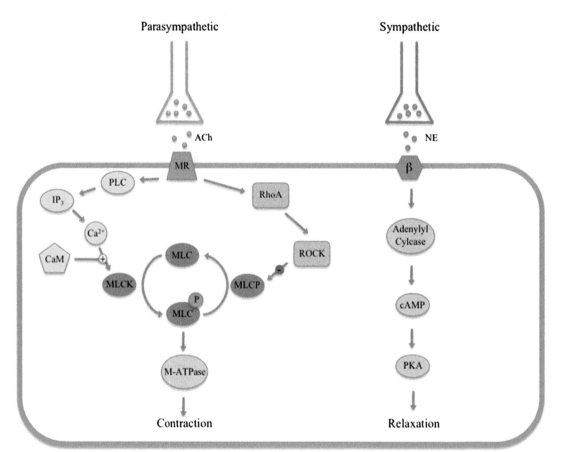

Detrusor Muscle Cell

Fig. 1. Parasympathetic and sympathetic innervation of bladder detrusor muscle. Acetylcholine (ACh) released by parasympathetic nerves binds to muscarinic receptors (MR), leading to the phosphorylation (P) of myosin regulatory light chain (MLC) through a pathway involving phospholipase C (PLC), inositol 1,4,5-triphosphate (IP_3), calcium (Ca^{2+}), calmodulin (CaM), and myosin light chain kinase (MLCK). Phosphorylated MLC activates myosin ATPase (M-ATPase) and initiates muscle contraction. Muscarinic receptors also regulate contraction through the RhoA/Rho-kinase pathway. RhoA activates Rho-kinase (ROCK), which inhibits myosin light chain phosphatase (MLCP). This action prevents MLCP from dephosphorylating activated MLC, allowing for continued contractions through MLC. Sympathetic nerves release norepinephrine (NE), which binds to β-adrenergic receptors (β), initiating a pathway leading to muscle relaxation through the mediators adenylyl cyclase, cyclic AMP (cAMP), and protein kinase A (PKA).

the mediator RhoA, a GTPase.[6] RhoA is regulated by various factors, including activation through muscarinic receptors.[7] Rho-kinase inhibits MLCP by phosphorylation, permitting continued activity of MLC in muscle contraction,[4] which indicates that the RhoA/Rho-kinase pathway allows for MLC activation at lower levels of calcium by inhibiting MLCP, known as calcium sensitivity.[8]

Bladder contraction and relaxation is also controlled by sympathetic innervation (see **Fig. 1**). There are 9 adrenergic receptor subtypes: 3 α_1, 3 α_2, and 3 β receptor subtypes.[9] Stimulation of β-adrenergic receptors by norepinephrine leads to detrusor muscle relaxation. The β_3 receptor subtype is the most abundantly expressed and seems to be the most important subtype for this interaction.[10–12] Signaling through the β receptor activates adenylyl cyclase to increase the levels cyclic AMP (cAMP).[13] Protein kinase A (PKA) is activated by cAMP, causing smooth muscle relaxation. In contrast, bladder outlet contraction is mainly under the control of α-adrenergic receptor stimulation by norepinephrine.[12] This occurs mainly through the α_{1A} subtype.[12,14,15] Activation of this receptor leads to G protein hydrolysis of IP$_3$. The resulting increase in intracellular calcium increases muscle tone in the bladder neck, urethra, and prostate.[12]

In animal models, NO has been shown to have a role in the regulation of smooth muscle tone in the bladder neck.[16,17] Recent evidence also indicates that NO may play a role in SMC relaxation in the human bladder neck.[18] NO is produced by NO synthases (NOS), of which 3 isoforms are known: neuronal NOS (nNOS), endothelial NOS (eNOS), and inducible NOS (iNOS).[19] The presence of NO leads to the production of cyclic guanosine monophosphate (cGMP) in SMCs. cGMP subsequently activates protein kinase G (PKG), initiating a phosphorylation cascade that ultimately leads to SMC relaxation.[20]

Prostate

The prostate is innervated by both the parasympathetic and sympathetic components of the ANS. Parasympathetic innervation helps to regulate the function of prostate epithelial cells through the activity of acetylcholine (ACh) on muscarinic receptors.[21] It seems that the M$_1$ subtype is most commonly associated with these epithelial cells.[22] There are also some data to suggest that a significantly smaller number of M$_2$ subtypes are found on stromal cells.[22] Animal models indicate that parasympathetic stimulation increases prostatic secretions mainly through activation of these epithelial M$_1$ receptors.[21,23]

Sympathetic innervation of the prostate is thought to be integral to the regulation of stromal cellular elements and may provide prostatic muscle tone. α-Adrenergic receptors are concentrated in the stromal cells and in prostatic blood vessels. Stromal cells express α_1 receptors, more specifically α_{1A}.[24,25] Given the sympathetic innervation to the stroma, sympathetic nerves play an important part in regulating prostatic SMC tone and help to coordinate prostatic secretion of fluid.[12] Prostatic SMC tone also seems to be regulated by the RhoA/Rho-kinase pathway. RhoA and Rho-kinase have been shown in human prostate tissue.[26] Inhibition of Rho-kinase in prostatic tissue by the inhibitor Y-27632 decreased norepinephrine-induced contraction at constant calcium concentration.[27]

Prostate growth is also influenced by autonomic neural input. This relationship has been well documented in various animal models. For example, McVary and colleagues[28] showed a positive association between the autonomic tone of the prostate and the rate of growth of the gland. Removal of this innervation is associated with a regression in prostate gland weight, DNA content, and protein content. These results support the notion that increased sympathetic input contributes to increased prostate growth and bladder outlet obstruction.

Nonadrenergic, noncholinergic neurotransmitters such as NO are also present in the prostate and seem to influence normal prostatic SMC tone and growth. nNOS and eNOS have been identified in the prostate by various methods. It seems that eNOS is localized to endothelial cells of the prostatic vessels.[29,30] In comparison, nNOS is concentrated around nerve terminals supplying stromal SMCs and glandular structures.[29–31]

Penis

The penis receives somatic, parasympathetic, and sympathetic efferent innervation. Somatic neural input to the bulbocavernosus and ischiocavernosus muscles improves penile rigidity and assists in expulsion of ejaculate.[32,33] Achieving tumescence involves interactions between the parasympathetic nerves and the vascular endothelial cells within the corpora cavernosa. NO is the mediator of this interaction.[34] Cavernosal nerves express the neuromodulator nNOS. NO is also produced by the local endothelial cells via eNOS. NO from both sources triggers the production of cGMP by cavernosal SMCs, ultimately leading to SMC relaxation and subsequent penile erection. The enzyme phosphodiesterase-5 (PDE-5) is responsible for cGMP degradation, which leads to detumescence. In addition, sympathetic neural input provides inhibition to parasympathetic neurons and also contributes to the relaxation of cavernosal SMCs. RhoA and Rho-kinase have also been identified in human penile tissues.[35,36] Inhibition of Rho-kinase by Y-27632 in rats receiving NOS inhibitors (ie, L-N^G-nitroarginine methyl ester hydrochloride [L-NAME]), showed an increase in intracavernosal pressure (ICP) that was independent of NO.[37] Likewise, ICP was increased after adeno-associated viral gene transfer of a dominant-negative RhoA mutant in rat penile tissue.[38] This indicates that the RhoA/Rho-kinase pathway regulates SMC contraction and maintenance of flaccidity. NO has been shown to inhibit the RhoA/Rho-kinase pathway in a crosstalk fashion.[39] Likewise, the RhoA/Rho-kinase pathway may also help to regulate NO signaling.[40]

ASSOCIATION OF AGE-RELATED CHANGES IN NEUROREGULATORY FACTORS WITH LUTS/BPH

LUTS secondary to BPH is a common age-related complaint. Various population-based studies have confirmed this association, and it has been estimated that BPH affects 50% of men aged 50 years or older and 90% of men aged 80 years or older.[41] BPH is a histologic definition that describes the

nodular proliferation of both the stromal and epithelial elements within the transition zone of the prostate.[42] LUTS secondary to BPH consists of both voiding and obstructive symptoms representing problems of bladder emptying and urine storage. Likewise, the prevalence of LUTS increases with age and it is found in 26% of men aged 40 to 50 years and 79% of men aged more than 70 years.[43] Although the exact cause of the development of LUTS/BPH in aging men is not yet fully understood, alterations in neuronal function secondary to aging processes, such as MSx and autonomic hyperactivity, and age-related changes in neuroregulatory pathways, such as NO and RhoA/Rho-kinase, seem to be major contributors to this process (**Fig. 2**).

MSx

MSx is a multifactorial disorder that has been associated with resistance to insulin-mediated glucose uptake.[44] However, the exact mechanisms leading to the development of this syndrome are currently unknown. The Adult Treatment Panel III defines this condition as meeting 3 or more of the following criteria: abdominal obesity with waist circumference greater than 102 cm, hypertriglyceridemia greater than 150 mg/dL, high-density lipoprotein (HDL) cholesterol less than 40 mg/dL, blood

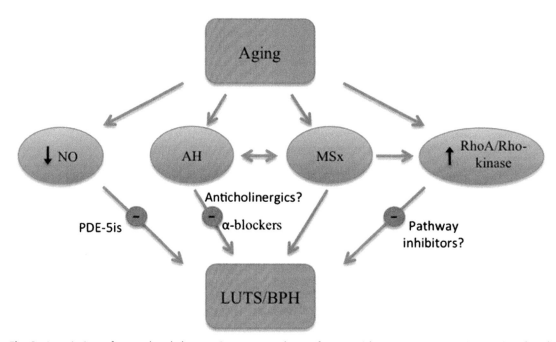

Fig. 2. Association of age-related changes in neuroregulatory factors with LUTS/BPH. Aging is associated with LUTS and BPH through decreased nitric oxide (NO) production, autonomic hyperactivity (AH), MSx, and upregulation of the RhoA/Rho-kinase pathway. The interactions of various pharmacologic treatments, such as phosphodiesterase-5 inhibitors (PDE-5is), anticholinergics, α-blockers, and, possibly in the future, RhoA/Rho-kinase pathway inhibitors, with this pathway are shown.

pressure greater than 135/85 mm Hg, and fasting plasma glucose greater than 110 mg/dL.[45] The prevalence of MSx has also been associated with age. MSx is found in 6.7% of those aged 20 to 29 years and increases to 42.0% of those aged 70 years or older.[46] Multiple studies have shown that men with the components of MSx have a significantly increased risk of LUTS/BPH, larger prostate volumes, and faster annual BPH growth rate.[47–54] In addition, it has been shown in animal models that long-term hyperglycemia causes neuronal cell death.[55] This apoptosis seems to favor parasympathetic rather than sympathetic neurons. Subsequent increased sympathetic tone, also known as autonomic hyperactivity, may contribute to the development of LUTS in MSx (discussed later).

Autonomic Hyperactivity

MSx may help explain the connection between alterations in neuronal function, aging, and autonomic hyperactivity. Aging has been associated with an overall increase in autonomic tone, and there is a positive association between age and levels of circulating norepinephrine. Autonomic hyperactivity is a component of MSx and involves dysregulation of parasympathetic and sympathetic tone. In addition, increased autonomic activity in aging rats has been associated with the development of prostatic hyperplasia.[28] Specifically, studies with spontaneously hypertensive rats showed that these rats were more likely to develop both increased autonomic activity and prostatic hyperplasia.[56] These rats voided more frequently, had increased sympathetic innervation to the bladder, and had more low-volume spontaneous bladder contractions.[57]

Epidemiologic studies have also elucidated the association between increased autonomic tone and BPH. Meigs and colleagues[58] showed that symptomatic BPH is more likely to be associated with sympathetic activation as approximated by increased serum markers of heart disease, increased β-blocker use, and sedentary lifestyle. McVary and colleagues[59] also examined markers of autonomic nervous system activity in men with LUTS secondary to BPH and International Prostate Symptom Scores (IPSS) of greater than or equal to 8. ANS activity was measured by heart rate, blood pressure, tilt table test response, and plasma and urinary catecholamines. There was a significant positive association between ANS hyperactivity and LUTS and prostate size. It seems that sympathetic nervous system tone contributes to the development of BPH in aging men.

NO

BPH has been associated with a decrease in the nitrinergic innervation of the prostate. The prostates of older rabbits were shown to have less NO-mediated relaxation and decreased overall nitrinergic innervation compared with younger counterparts.[60] Bloch and colleagues[30] examined prostatic tissue of men with symptomatic BPH and found a qualitatively decreased density of nitrogenic nerves compared with controls by measuring nicotinamide adenine dinucleotide phosphate diaphorase (NADPH-d), a marker for NOS expression. Similarly, it has been shown that there is decreased expression of the NOS gene in transurethral resection of prostate tissue samples of men with BPH compared with normal prostate tissue.[61] The results of this study suggest that older men and those with larger prostates had significantly less NOS expression then younger men with smaller prostates.

RhoA/Rho-Kinase

Given its role in the regulation of muscle activity in both the bladder and prostate, it is likely that age-related alterations in this system could contribute to the development of urinary symptoms. The RhoA/Rho-kinase pathway may contribute to the development of LUTS/BPH, because inhibition of Rho-kinase prevents noradrenergic-induced contractions and proliferation of prostate SMCs.[26] This bladder outlet obstruction caused by SMC proliferation may cause hypertrophy of the bladder and worsening of urinary symptoms. Support from this is derived from the increased RhoA and Rho-kinase expression and decreased MLCP activity in hypertrophied bladders.[62] In addition, rat bladders that were denervated and hypertrophied, but not obstructed, showed that the effect of a muscarinic agonist was decreased by Rho-kinase inhibition.[63] However, in normal bladders, Rho-kinase inhibition reduced the potency of carbachol but did not affect maximal contraction.[64] Diabetes has also been shown to affect the RhoA/Rho-kinase pathway in the bladder. Animal models with diabetic rabbits show higher Rho-kinase expression, increased MLC phosphorylation, and decreased effectiveness of the Rho-kinase inhibitor Y-27632 on levels of MLC phosphorylation in the bladder.[65,66] Taken together, these data suggest that the imbalance in the RhoA/Rho-kinase pathway may also influence LUTS.

TREATMENT OF LUTS/BPH

The importance of neuronal influences on the development of LUTS/BPH is underscored by the various therapeutic strategies that target them. These interventions include α-adrenergic antagonists, anticholinergics, and PDE-5 inhibitors (PDE-5i).

α-Adrenergic Antagonists

Modulation of autonomic activity by α-receptor antagonism has shown benefit in the treatment of LUTS/BPH. The inhibition of adrenergic receptors seems to decrease SMC tone in the bladder and prostate, decrease the number of SMCs, and improve LUTS related to BPH.[67] It is unclear whether these drugs primarily produce their benefit through a direct effect on the prostate and bladder or through indirect effects via the central nervous system. Both first-generation agents (eg, phenoxybenzamine) and second-generation agents (eg, prazosin, terazosin, doxazosin, and alfuzosin) have been well studied with favorable improvements in IPSS scores and urinary flow rates.[67] This suggests a prominent role of autonomic activity in LUTS/BPH.

Anticholinergics

Traditionally, anticholinergics were contraindicated in LUTS secondary to BPH because of concern about the risk of developing acute urinary retention (AUR). However, anticholinergics have been shown to be safe in men with LUTS.[68] Although anticholinergics improve the symptoms of urgency and frequency, the effectiveness of these medications in the treatment of primarily obstructive symptoms has not been clearly shown.[67,68] In addition, some studies have examined the role of cholinergic neuromodulation in the development of LUTS in aging men from studying the effects of botulinum toxin. Specifically, botulinum neurotoxin prevents the presynaptic release of ACh.[69] By blocking the release of ACh, this intervention acts to chemically remove cholinergic input. Many studies have shown improvement in LUTS after intraprostatic botulinum injections.[70–74] However, large, randomized, placebo-controlled studies are needed to confirm these results. Taken together, these studies suggest that cholinergic innervation may contribute to prostate growth and the development of LUTS, but future research is required.

PDE-5 Inhibitors and NO

Decreased nitrinergic innervation and NOS expression in the aging prostate suggest that the NO pathway may also contribute to the development of LUTS secondary to BPH. Studies have shown that targeting this pathway improves LUTS. For example, Klotz and colleagues[75]

showed in an open-labeled trial that isosorbide dinitrate in patients with heart disease and LUTS improves IPSS, decreased peripheral vascular resistance, and increase in peak flow rates.

Subsequent studies examined the effects of PDE-5 inhibitors (PDE-5i) on LUTS/BPH. These pharmacologic agents work by preventing the degradation of cGMP by PDE-5, leading to improved SMC relaxation.[76] Several studies have also shown that sildenafil, a PDE-5i, improves LUTS. For example, McVary and colleagues[77] examined the effects of sildenafil in men with ED and LUTS in a randomized, double-blind, placebo-controlled trial. Men treated with a 12-week course of the drug experienced a mean decrease in IPSS of 6.32 compared with a decrease of 1.93 in the placebo group. McVary and colleagues[78] also examined the effects of tadalafil in a randomized, double-blind, placebo-controlled trial in 281 men with moderate to severe LUTS. At 6 weeks, the treatment group showed a significant mean change in IPSS score of −2.8 compared with −1.2 in the placebo group.

Similarly, Kaplan and colleagues[79] showed the efficacy of combination sildenafil and alfuzosin in men suffering from LUTS and ED in an open-labeled study. The combination group had the greatest improvement in IPSS score from an initial mean of 17.8 (± 4.7) to 13.5 (± 4.2), representing a −24.1% change, compared with a change of 17.3 (± 4.3) to 14.6 (± 3.7) in the alfuzosin group and 16.9 (± 4.1) to 14.9 (± 4.2) in the sildenafil groups, representing decreases of 15.6% and 16.9% respectively. The ability of PDE-5is to improve LUTS suggests that the NO pathway contributes to the development of LUTS in aging men.

ASSOCIATION OF AGE-RELATED CHANGES IN NEUROREGULATORY FACTORS WITH ED

The effects of aging on the nervous system's interactions with the penis are most easily seen in the pathogenesis of ED. There is a clear association of ED with age in multiple epidemiologic studies. In the Massachusetts Male Aging Study, the prevalence of ED increased from 52% in men aged 40 to 70 years to 70% in men aged 70 years or older.[80] There are various causes linked to the development of ED, including psychogenic, endocrinologic, drug-induced, vasculogenic, and neurogenic causes. Well-known neurologic causes include Parkinson disease, stroke, and spinal cord injuries. Various neuroregulatory changes that occur in aging men have also been associated with decline in erectile function. These changes are associated with MSx, autonomic hyperactivity, alterations in the regulation of the NO, hypogonadism, and changes in the RhoA/Rho-kinase pathway (**Fig. 3**). Currently available treatment of ED, such as PDE-5is and testosterone in hypogonadal men, underscore the importance of age-related changes in the neuroregulation of ED.

MSx and Autonomic Hyperactivity

There is a high rate of sexual dysfunction in aging men with MSx. Corona and colleagues[81] discovered that, in a group of 236 men with MSx, 96.5% reported having ED. MSx has been associated with a significantly decreased International Index of Erectile Function (IIEF) score. There is also some evidence to support the role of autonomic hyperactivity in ED. Specifically, spontaneously hypertensive rates show increased autonomic activity and ED.[82] However, of all the components of MSx, it was noted by Corona and colleagues[81] that abnormal fasting plasma glucose was the most significant factor associated with the development of ED. Hyperglycemia can have a negative impact on cavernosal nerve function and, as

a result, erectile function.[83] The contribution of hyperglycemia/diabetes to ED is multifactorial but involves the dysregulation of NO signaling.

NO

Because erectile function is heavily dependent on NO, it is reasonable to hypothesize that alterations in the NO pathway may also contribute to the development of ED. In aging men, changes in the NO pathway have been most closely associated with the development of diabetes and hypogonadism. For example, diabetic rat models have shown that there is a selective and significant degeneration of penile NO-producing neurons compared with healthy animal controls.[55] In addition, diabetes has been associated with a decrease in the expression of neuronal NOS.[84] Studies with rats have shown an association between decreased neuronal NO expression and diabetes. Research using tissues obtained from diabetic humans has confirmed that diabetics have decreased NOS activity.[85] The downstream pathways of NO signaling are also negatively affected in diabetes.

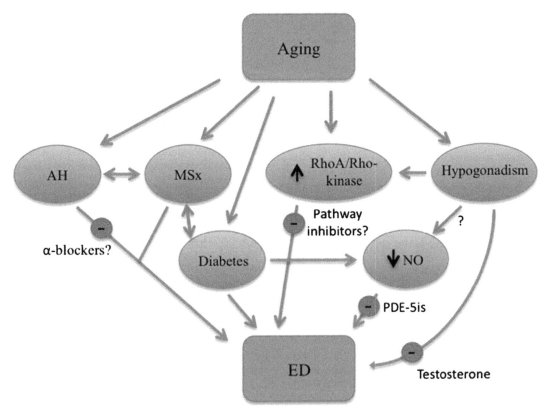

Fig. 3. Association of age-related changes in neuroregulatory factors with ED. Aging is associated with ED through AH, MSx, diabetes, upregulation of the RhoA/Rho-kinase pathway, hypogonadism, and decreased NO production. The interactions of various pharmacologic treatments of ED, such as phosphodiesterase-5 inhibitors (PDE-5is) and testosterone, with this pathway are shown. Also included are less supported or potential future treatments, such as α-blockers and RhoA/Rho-kinase pathway inhibitors.

For example, diabetes may negatively affect guanylyl cyclase.[86] Taken together, it seems that aging and its associated comorbidities influence the NO pathway. These alterations most likely influence penile tumescence and the onset of ED.

Hypogonadism

In addition to diabetes, hypogonadism has been associated with dysregulation of the NO pathway and the development of ED. As men age, there is an overall decrease in testosterone levels. This decrease was shown in the Baltimore Longitudinal Study on Aging, which showed that, as men age after their 30s, there is an associated 1% yearly decrease in total serum testosterone levels.[87] Low total and bioavailable testosterone has been associated with poor erectile function.[88] This association has been appreciated in studies examining the erectile function in castrated animals. A decline in erectile function along with a disruption in the structure and function of the cavernosal nerve has been shown in castrated animals.[89,90] More importantly, the observed structural changes were reversed when the animals were treated with testosterone.[89]

The production of NO is influenced by testosterone exposure through regulation of corpus cavernosum NOS isoform expression.[91] Studies with castrated animals have also shown that testosterone can restore NOS activity and erections.[89,91,92] In addition, testosterone has been show to be important in regulating the production of PDE-5. Castrated animals have decreased levels of PDE-5 that are improved with testosterone.[93–95] However, treatment with PDE-5 inhibitors in castrated animals did not show a significant increase in ICP after pelvic nerve stimulation.[94] Traish and colleagues[91] noted that this dual role of androgens in the upregulation of both NOS and PDE-5, although contradictory, may suggest a homeostatic function of androgens in the NO pathway. Intuitively, an age-related decline in androgens would cause a disruption of this homeostasis.

RhoA/Rho-Kinase

The Rho-kinase pathway also seems to affect erectile function in aging men. Rajasekaran and colleagues[96] showed that inhibition of the RhoA/Rho-kinase pathway by Y-27632 improved electrically stimulated erectile responses in aged rats. Subsequently, it was shown that inhibition of this pathway in aged rates improved erectile responses more in older rats.[97] There is an increased imbalance between nNOS and Rho-kinase protein expression in aged rats, and these older rats had greater improvement in erectile function after Y-27632 inhibition.[98] Diabetic rats have shown increased RhoA/Rho-kinase pathway proteins in penile tissue and improved erectile response to Y-27632.[40,99] There is also a growing body of evidence that hypogonadism may contribute to ED through the RhoA/Rho-kinase pathway. Castrated rats showed increased expression of RhoA and Rho-kinase in penile tissue and an increased contractile response to phenylephrine that was reversed with Rho-kinase inhibition.[100]

TREATMENT OF ED

As with LUTS secondary to BPH, the pharmacologic treatment of ED highlights the importance of changes in the neuroregulatory pathways controlling erectile dysfunction in aging men. The primary oral medical treatment of ED is the PDE-5i class of drugs. Currently, there are 3 available drugs within this class: sildenafil, vardenafil, and tadalafil. All of these agents work on the NO pathway by inhibiting PDE-5, preventing the degradation of cGMP, and leading to improved corporal SMC relaxation.[76] These drugs have shown improvement in ED in aged men with and without comorbidities. For example, tadalafil showed a mean improvement in IIEF scores of 8.8 points at 12 weeks in men more than 65 years of age without comorbidities such as diabetes.[101] PDE-5i has also shown improvement in ED in men with MSx, albeit not as robust as in men without these comorbidities. Specifically, men with 4 components for MSx showed a 20% response to sildenafil compared with 90% of men with none of the components.[102] The overall decreased response in men with MSx indicates that the associated neurologic changes in NO regulation are only 1 mechanism in the pathogenesis of ED.

Although PDE-5i intervention is the mainstay of current medical management of ED, other therapies may be of benefit in certain populations. Testosterone can help improve erectile function in hypogonadal men.[103] In addition, α-blockers have shown some benefit in improving erectile function in certain scenarios, such as in men with MSx or in combination with a PDE-5i.[104,105] However, it is unclear whether this benefit is derived from the improvement in LUTS/BPH that is often associated with ED. RhoA/Rho-kinase pathway inhibitors may be potential future treatments for both ED and LUTS/BPH, but currently there are none approved for clinical use.

SUMMARY

Aging men are subject to the development of LUTS/BPH and ED. Various factors have been shown to contribute to the pathogenesis of both of these conditions, including changes in the innervation and neuroregulatory pathways of the lower urinary tract. LUTS/BPH and ED in aging men are affected by alterations in neuronal function secondary to aging processes, such as MSx and autonomic hyperactivity. In addition, age-related changes in neuroregulatory pathways such as NO and RhoA/Rho-kinase have also been shown to contribute to the pathogenesis of these conditions. Various pharmacologic agents that target these pathways, such as α-blockers and PDE-5is, underscore the contribution of neuroregulatory factors to the development of LUTS/BPH and ED.

REFERENCES

1. Caulfield MP, Birdsall NJ. International Union of Pharmacology. XVII. Classification of muscarinic acetylcholine receptors. Pharmacol Rev 1998; 50(2):279–90.
2. Abrams P, Andersson KE, Buccafusco JJ, et al. Muscarinic receptors: their distribution and function in body systems, and the implications for treating overactive bladder. Br J Pharmacol 2006; 148(5):565–78.
3. Hegde SS. Muscarinic receptors in the bladder: from basic research to therapeutics. Br J Pharmacol 2006;147(Suppl 2):S80–7.
4. Somlyo AP, Somlyo AV. Signal transduction by G-proteins, rho-kinase and protein phosphatase to smooth muscle and non-muscle myosin II. J Physiol 2000;522(Pt 2):177–85.
5. Kimura K, Ito M, Amano M, et al. Regulation of myosin phosphatase by Rho and Rho-associated kinase (Rho-kinase). Science 1996;273(5272): 245–8.
6. Wettschureck N, Offermanns S. Rho/Rho-kinase mediated signaling in physiology and pathophysiology. J Mol Med 2002;80(10):629–38.
7. Peters SL, Schmidt M, Michel MC. Rho kinase: a target for treating urinary bladder dysfunction? Trends Pharmacol Sci 2006;27(9):492–7.
8. Christ GJ, Andersson KE. Rho-kinase and effects of Rho-kinase inhibition on the lower urinary tract. Neurourol Urodyn 2007;26(Suppl 6):948–54.
9. Hieble JP, Bylund DB, Clarke DE, et al. International Union of Pharmacology. X. Recommendation for nomenclature of alpha 1-adrenoceptors: consensus update. Pharmacol Rev 1995;47(2):267–70.
10. Fujimura T, Tamura K, Tsutsumi T, et al. Expression and possible functional role of the beta3-adrenoceptor in human and rat detrusor muscle. J Urol 1999;161(2):680–5.
11. Seguchi H, Nishimura J, Zhou Y, et al. Expression of beta3-adrenoceptors in rat detrusor smooth muscle. J Urol 1998;159(6):2197–201.
12. Michel MC, Vrydag W. Alpha1-, alpha2- and beta-adrenoceptors in the urinary bladder, urethra and prostate. Br J Pharmacol 2006;147(Suppl 2):S88–119.
13. Bylund JE, Zhang L, Haines MA, et al. Analysis by fluorescence microscopy of the development of compartment-specific gene expression during sporulation of Bacillus subtilis. J Bacteriol 1994; 176(10):2898–905.
14. Nasu K, Moriyama N, Fukasawa R, et al. Quantification and distribution of alpha1-adrenoceptor subtype mRNAs in human proximal urethra. Br J Pharmacol 1998;123(7):1289–93.
15. Nasu K, Moriyama N, Kawabe K, et al. Quantification and distribution of alpha 1-adrenoceptor subtype mRNAs in human prostate: comparison of benign hypertrophied tissue and non-hypertrophied tissue. Br J Pharmacol 1996;119(5):797–803.
16. Hernandez M, Recio P, Barahona MV, et al. Prejunctional alpha2-adrenoceptors modulation of the nitrergic transmission in the pig urinary bladder neck. Neurourol Urodyn 2007;26(4):578–83.
17. Hernandez M, Barahona MV, Recio P, et al. Role of neuronal voltage-gated K(+) channels in the modulation of the nitrergic neurotransmission of the pig urinary bladder neck. Br J Pharmacol 2008;153(6):1251–8.
18. Bustamante S, Orensanz LM, Recio P, et al. Functional evidence of nitrergic neurotransmission in the human urinary bladder neck. Neurosci Lett 2010;477(2):91–4.
19. Forstermann U, Closs EI, Pollock JS, et al. Nitric oxide synthase isozymes. Characterization, purification, molecular cloning, and functions. Hypertension 1994;23(6 Pt 2):1121–31.
20. Carvajal JA, Germain AM, Huidobro-Toro JP, et al. Molecular mechanism of cGMP-mediated smooth muscle relaxation. J Cell Physiol 2000;184(3): 409–20.
21. Ventura S, Pennefather J, Mitchelson F. Cholinergic innervation and function in the prostate gland. Pharmacol Ther 2002;94(1–2):93–112.
22. Ruggieri MR, Colton MD, Wang P, et al. Human prostate muscarinic receptor subtypes. J Pharmacol Exp Ther 1995;274(2):976–82.
23. Wang JM, McKenna KE, Lee C. Determination of prostatic secretion in rats: effect of neurotransmitters and testosterone. Prostate 1991;18(4):289–301.
24. Kobayashi S, Tang R, Shapiro E, et al. Characterization and localization of prostatic alpha 1 adrenoceptors using radioligand receptor binding on slide-mounted tissue section. J Urol 1993;150(6): 2002–6.
25. Price DT, Schwinn DA, Lomasney JW, et al. Identification, quantification, and localization of mRNA for three distinct alpha 1 adrenergic receptor subtypes in human prostate. J Urol 1993;150(2 Pt 1): 546–51.

26. Rees RW, Foxwell NA, Ralph DJ, et al. Y-27632, a Rho-kinase inhibitor, inhibits proliferation and adrenergic contraction of prostatic smooth muscle cells. J Urol 2003;170(6 Pt 1):2517–22.

27. Takahashi R, Nishimura J, Seki N, et al. RhoA/Rho kinase-mediated Ca2+ sensitization in the contraction of human prostate. Neurourol Urodyn 2007; 26(4):547–51.

28. McVary KT, Razzaq A, Lee C, et al. Growth of the rat prostate gland is facilitated by the autonomic nervous system. Biol Reprod 1994;51(1):99–107.

29. Gradini R, Realacci M, Ginepri A, et al. Nitric oxide synthases in normal and benign hyperplastic human prostate: immunohistochemistry and molecular biology. J Pathol 1999;189(2):224–9.

30. Bloch W, Klotz T, Loch C, et al. Distribution of nitric oxide synthase implies a regulation of circulation, smooth muscle tone, and secretory function in the human prostate by nitric oxide. Prostate 1997; 33(1):1–8.

31. Burnett AL, Maguire MP, Chamness SL, et al. Characterization and localization of nitric oxide synthase in the human prostate. Urology 1995;45(3):435–9.

32. Schmidt MH, Schmidt HS. The ischiocavernosus and bulbospongiosus muscles in mammalian penile rigidity. Sleep 1993;16(2):171–83.

33. Giuliano F, Rampin O. Neural control of erection. Physiol Behav 2004;83(2):189–201.

34. Burnett AL. Role of nitric oxide in the physiology of erection. Biol Reprod 1995;52(3):485–9.

35. Rees RW, Ziessen T, Ralph DJ, et al. Human and rabbit cavernosal smooth muscle cells express Rho-kinase. Int J Impot Res 2002;14(1):1–7.

36. Wang H, Eto M, Steers WD, et al. RhoA-mediated Ca2+ sensitization in erectile function. J Biol Chem 2002;277(34):30614–21.

37. Chitaley K, Wingard CJ, Clinton Webb R, et al. Antagonism of Rho-kinase stimulates rat penile erection via a nitric oxide-independent pathway. Nat Med 2001;7(1):119–22.

38. Chitaley K, Bivalacqua TJ, Champion HC, et al. Adeno-associated viral gene transfer of dominant negative RhoA enhances erectile function in rats. Biochem Biophys Res Commun 2002;298(3):427–32.

39. Mills TM, Chitaley K, Lewis RW, et al. Nitric oxide inhibits RhoA/Rho-kinase signaling to cause penile erection. Eur J Pharmacol 2002;439(1–3): 173–4.

40. Bivalacqua TJ, Champion HC, Usta MF, et al. RhoA/Rho-kinase suppresses endothelial nitric oxide synthase in the penis: a mechanism for diabetes-associated erectile dysfunction. Proc Natl Acad Sci U S A 2004;101(24):9121–6.

41. Rosen R, Altwein J, Boyle P, et al. Lower urinary tract symptoms and male sexual dysfunction: the Multinational Survey of the Aging Male (MSAM-7). Eur Urol 2003;44(6):637–49.

42. Lee C, Kozlowski JM, Grayhack JT. Etiology of benign prostatic hyperplasia. Urol Clin North Am 1995;22(2):237–46.

43. Guess HA, Arrighi HM, Metter EJ, et al. Cumulative prevalence of prostatism matches the autopsy prevalence of benign prostatic hyperplasia. Prostate 1990;17(3):241–6.

44. Hammarsten J, Hogstedt B. Hyperinsulinaemia as a risk factor for developing benign prostatic hyperplasia. Eur Urol 2001;39(2):151–8.

45. National Cholesterol Education Program (NCEP) Expert Panel on Detection, Evaluation, and Treatment of High Blood Cholesterol in Adults (Adult Treatment Panel III). Third Report of the National Cholesterol Education Program (NCEP) Expert Panel on Detection, Evaluation, and Treatment of High Blood Cholesterol in Adults (Adult Treatment Panel III) final report. Circulation 2002;106(25):3143–421.

46. Ford ES, Giles WH, Dietz WH. Prevalence of the metabolic syndrome among US adults: findings from the third National Health and Nutrition Examination Survey. JAMA 2002;287(3):356–9.

47. Glynn RJ, Campion EW, Bouchard GR, et al. The development of benign prostatic hyperplasia among volunteers in the Normative Aging Study. Am J Epidemiol 1985;121(1):78–90.

48. Hammarsten J, Hogstedt B, Holthuis N, et al. Components of the metabolic syndrome-risk factors for the development of benign prostatic hyperplasia. Prostate Cancer Prostatic Dis 1998; 1(3):157–62.

49. Hammarsten J, Hogstedt B. Clinical, anthropometric, metabolic and insulin profile of men with fast annual growth rates of benign prostatic hyperplasia. Blood Press 1999;8(1):29–36.

50. Rohrmann S, Smit E, Giovannucci E, et al. Associations of obesity with lower urinary tract symptoms and noncancer prostate surgery in the Third National Health and Nutrition Examination Survey. Am J Epidemiol 2004;159(4):390–7.

51. Parsons JK, Carter HB, Partin AW, et al. Metabolic factors associated with benign prostatic hyperplasia. J Clin Endocrinol Metab 2006; 91(7):2562–8.

52. Seim A, Hoyo C, Ostbye T, et al. The prevalence and correlates of urinary tract symptoms in Norwegian men: the HUNT study. BJU Int 2005;96(1):88–92.

53. Laven BA, Orsini N, Andersson SO, et al. Birth weight, abdominal obesity and the risk of lower urinary tract symptoms in a population based study of Swedish men. J Urol 2008;179(5):1891–5 [discussion: 1895–6].

54. Kristal AR, Arnold KB, Schenk JM, et al. Race/ethnicity, obesity, health related behaviors and the risk of symptomatic benign prostatic hyperplasia: results from the prostate cancer prevention trial. J Urol 2007;177(4):1395–400 [quiz: 1591].

55. Cellek S, Rodrigo J, Lobos E, et al. Selective nitrergic neurodegeneration in diabetes mellitus - a nitric oxide-dependent phenomenon. Br J Pharmacol 1999;128(8):1804–12.
56. Persson K, Pandita RK, Spitsbergen JM, et al. Spinal and peripheral mechanisms contributing to hyperactive voiding in spontaneously hypertensive rats. Am J Physiol 1998;275(4 Pt 2):R1366–73.
57. Steers WD, Clemow DB, Persson K, et al. The spontaneously hypertensive rat: insight into the pathogenesis of irritative symptoms in benign prostatic hyperplasia and young anxious males. Exp Physiol 1999;84(1):137–47.
58. Meigs JB, Mohr B, Barry MJ, et al. Risk factors for clinical benign prostatic hyperplasia in a community-based population of healthy aging men. J Clin Epidemiol 2001;54(9):935–44.
59. McVary KT, Rademaker A, Lloyd GL, et al. Autonomic nervous system overactivity in men with lower urinary tract symptoms secondary to benign prostatic hyperplasia. J Urol 2005;174(4 Pt 1):1327–433.
60. Aikawa K, Yokota T, Okamura H, et al. Endogenous nitric oxide-mediated relaxation and nitrinergic innervation in the rabbit prostate: the changes with aging. Prostate 2001;48(1):40–6.
61. Luo J, Dunn T, Ewing C, et al. Gene expression signature of benign prostatic hyperplasia revealed by cDNA microarray analysis. Prostate 2002;51(3):189–200.
62. Bing W, Chang S, Hypolite JA, et al. Obstruction-induced changes in urinary bladder smooth muscle contractility: a role for Rho kinase. Am J Physiol Renal Physiol 2003;285(5):F990–7.
63. Braverman AS, Doumanian LR, Ruggieri MR, et al. M2 and M3 muscarinic receptor activation of urinary bladder contractile signal transduction. II. Denervated rat bladder. J Pharmacol Exp Ther 2006;316(2):875–80.
64. Braverman AS, Tibb AS, Ruggieri MR Sr. M2 and M3 muscarinic receptor activation of urinary bladder contractile signal transduction. I. Normal rat bladder. J Pharmacol Exp Ther 2006;316(2):869–74.
65. Chang S, Hypolite JA, DiSanto ME, et al. Increased basal phosphorylation of detrusor smooth muscle myosin in alloxan-induced diabetic rabbit is mediated by upregulation of Rho-kinase beta and CPI-17. Am J Physiol Renal Physiol 2006;290(3):F650–6.
66. Su X, Changolkar A, Chacko S, et al. Diabetes decreases rabbit bladder smooth muscle contraction while increasing levels of myosin light chain phosphorylation. Am J Physiol Renal Physiol 2004;287(4):F690–9.
67. Auffenberg GB, Helfand BT, McVary KT. Established medical therapy for benign prostatic hyperplasia. Urol Clin North Am 2009;36(4):443–59, v–vi.
68. Blake-James BT, Rashidian A, Ikeda Y, et al. The role of anticholinergics in men with lower urinary tract symptoms suggestive of benign prostatic hyperplasia: a systematic review and meta-analysis. BJU Int 2007;99(1):85–96.
69. Pellizzari R, Rossetto O, Schiavo G, et al. Tetanus and botulinum neurotoxins: mechanism of action and therapeutic uses. Philos Trans R Soc Lond B Biol Sci 1999;354(1381):259–68.
70. Maria G, Brisinda G, Civello IM, et al. Relief by botulinum toxin of voiding dysfunction due to benign prostatic hyperplasia: results of a randomized, placebo-controlled study. Urology 2003;62(2):259–64 [discussion: 264–5].
71. Chuang YC, Chiang PH, Huang CC, et al. Botulinum toxin type A improves benign prostatic hyperplasia symptoms in patients with small prostates. Urology 2005;66(4):775–9.
72. Chuang YC, Chiang PH, Yoshimura N, et al. Sustained beneficial effects of intraprostatic botulinum toxin type A on lower urinary tract symptoms and quality of life in men with benign prostatic hyperplasia. BJU Int 2006;98(5):1033–7 [discussion: 1337].
73. Nikoobakht M, Daneshpajooh A, Ahmadi H, et al. Intraprostatic botulinum toxin type A injection for the treatment of benign prostatic hyperplasia: initial experience with Dysport. Scand J Urol Nephrol 2010;44(3):151–7.
74. Chen JL, Chen CY, Kuo HC. Botulinum toxin A injection to the bladder neck and urethra for medically refractory lower urinary tract symptoms in men without prostatic obstruction. J Formos Med Assoc 2009;108(12):950–6.
75. Klotz T, Mathers MJ, Bloch W, et al. Nitric oxide based influence of nitrates on micturition in patients with benign prostatic hyperplasia. Int Urol Nephrol 1999;31(3):335–41.
76. Lue TF. Erectile dysfunction. N Engl J Med 2000;342(24):1802–13.
77. McVary KT, Monnig W, Camps JL Jr, et al. Sildenafil citrate improves erectile function and urinary symptoms in men with erectile dysfunction and lower urinary tract symptoms associated with benign prostatic hyperplasia: a randomized, double-blind trial. J Urol 2007;177(3):1071–7.
78. McVary KT, Roehrborn CG, Kaminetsky JC, et al. Tadalafil relieves lower urinary tract symptoms secondary to benign prostatic hyperplasia. J Urol 2007;177(4):1401–7.
79. Kaplan SA, Gonzalez RR, Te AE. Combination of alfuzosin and sildenafil is superior to monotherapy in treating lower urinary tract symptoms and erectile dysfunction. Eur Urol 2007;51(6):1717–23.
80. Feldman HA, Goldstein I, Hatzichristou DG, et al. Impotence and its medical and psychosocial correlates: results of the Massachusetts Male Aging Study. J Urol 1994;151(1):54–61.

81. Corona G, Mannucci E, Schulman C, et al. Psychobiologic correlates of the metabolic syndrome and associated sexual dysfunction. Eur Urol Sep 2006; 50(3):595–604 [discussion: 604].

82. Hale TM, Okabe H, Bushfield TL, et al. Recovery of erectile function after brief aggressive antihypertensive therapy. J Urol 2002;168(1):348–54.

83. Hecht MJ, Neundorfer B, Kiesewetter F, et al. Neuropathy is a major contributing factor to diabetic erectile dysfunction. Neurol Res 2001;23(6):651–4.

84. Vernet D, Cai L, Garban H, et al. Reduction of penile nitric oxide synthase in diabetic BB/WORdp (type I) and BBZ/WORdp (type II) rats with erectile dysfunction. Endocrinology 1995; 136(12):5709–17.

85. Tuncayengin A, Biri H, Onaran M, et al. Cavernosal tissue nitrite, nitrate, malondialdehyde and glutathione levels in diabetic and non-diabetic erectile dysfunction. Int J Androl 2003;26(4):250–4.

86. Seftel AD, Vaziri ND, Ni Z, et al. Advanced glycation end products in human penis: elevation in diabetic tissue, site of deposition, and possible effect through iNOS or eNOS. Urology 1997; 50(6):1016–26.

87. Harman SM, Metter EJ, Tobin JD, et al. Longitudinal effects of aging on serum total and free testosterone levels in healthy men. Baltimore Longitudinal Study of Aging. J Clin Endocrinol Metab 2001; 86(2):724–31.

88. Kratzik CW, Schatzl G, Lunglmayr G, et al. The impact of age, body mass index and testosterone on erectile dysfunction. J Urol 2005; 174(1):240–3.

89. Rogers RS, Graziottin TM, Lin CS, et al. Intracavernosal vascular endothelial growth factor (VEGF) injection and adeno-associated virus-mediated VEGF gene therapy prevent and reverse venogenic erectile dysfunction in rats. Int J Impot Res 2003;15(1):26–37.

90. Keast JR, Gleeson RJ, Shulkes A, et al. Maturational and maintenance effects of testosterone on terminal axon density and neuropeptide expression in the rat vas deferens. Neuroscience 2002; 112(2):391–8.

91. Traish AM, Goldstein I, Kim NN. Testosterone and erectile function: from basic research to a new clinical paradigm for managing men with androgen insufficiency and erectile dysfunction. Eur Urol 2007;52(1):54–70.

92. Zvara P, Sioufi R, Schipper HM, et al. Nitric oxide mediated erectile activity is a testosterone dependent event: a rat erection model. Int J Impot Res 1995;7(4):209–19.

93. Armagan A, Kim NN, Goldstein I, et al. Dose-response relationship between testosterone and erectile function: evidence for the existence of a critical threshold. J Androl 2006;27(4):517–26.

94. Zhang XH, Morelli A, Luconi M, et al. Testosterone regulates PDE5 expression and in vivo responsiveness to tadalafil in rat corpus cavernosum. Eur Urol 2005;47(3):409–16 [discussion: 416].

95. Morelli A, Filippi S, Mancina R, et al. Androgens regulate phosphodiesterase type 5 expression and functional activity in corpora cavernosa. Endocrinology 2004;145(5):2253–63.

96. Rajasekaran M, Kasyan A, Jain A, et al. Altered growth factor expression in the aging penis: the Brown-Norway rat model. J Androl 2002;23(3):393–9.

97. Jin L, Liu T, Lagoda GA, et al. Elevated RhoA/Rho-kinase activity in the aged rat penis: mechanism for age-associated erectile dysfunction. FASEB J 2006;20(3):536–8.

98. Gao BH, Zhao ST, Meng FW, et al. Y-27632 improves the erectile dysfunction with ageing in SD rats through adjusting the imbalance between nNo and the Rho-kinase pathways. Andrologia 2007;39(4):146–50.

99. Chang S, Hypolite JA, Changolkar A, et al. Increased contractility of diabetic rabbit corpora smooth muscle in response to endothelin is mediated via Rho-kinase beta. Int J Impot Res 2003;15(1):53–62.

100. Wingard CJ, Johnson JA, Holmes A, et al. Improved erectile function after Rho-kinase inhibition in a rat castrate model of erectile dysfunction. Am J Physiol Regul Integr Comp Physiol 2003; 284(6):R1572–9.

101. Sharlip ID, Shumaker BP, Hakim LS, et al. Tadalafil is efficacious and well tolerated in the treatment of erectile dysfunction (ED) in men over 65 years of age: results from Multiple Observations in Men with ED in National Tadalafil Study in the United States. J Sex Med 2008;5(3):716–25.

102. Suetomi T, Kawai K, Hinotsu S, et al. Negative impact of metabolic syndrome on the responsiveness to sildenafil in Japanese men. J Sex Med 2008;5(6):1443–50.

103. Jain P, Rademaker AW, McVary KT. Testosterone supplementation for erectile dysfunction: results of a meta-analysis. J Urol 2000;164(2):371–5.

104. Kumar R, Nehra A, Jacobson DJ, et al. Alpha-blocker use is associated with decreased risk of sexual dysfunction. Urology 2009;74(1):82–7.

105. Oger S, Behr-Roussel D, Gorny D, et al. Combination of doxazosin and sildenafil exerts an additive relaxing effect compared with each compound alone on human cavernosal and prostatic tissue. J Sex Med 2009;6(3):836–47.

The Optimal Male Health Diet and Dietary Supplement Program

Mark A. Moyad, MD, MPH[a,b,*]

KEYWORDS

- Men • Diet • Cardiovascular disease • Dietary supplements

Before recommending the optimal male diet, male health concerns need to be triaged. Reiterating the most common causes of morbidity and mortality allows for an easier understanding of dietary and supplement changes that should be recommended for men in general. These recommendations need to be simple, logical, and practical for the patient as well as the clinician. Thus, reviewing common causes of mortality is paramount to construing all other recommendations in this article.

Cardiovascular disease (CVD) is the number 1 overall cause of mortality in the United States and in other industrialized countries.[1–3] CVD is currently the number 1 cause of death worldwide, and is the number 1 cause of death in every region of the world with the exception of sub-Saharan Africa. Cancer is the second leading cause of death in the United States and in most developed countries, and is expected to mirror the number of deaths from CVD in the next several years in various regions of the world. CVD has been the number 1 cause of death in the United States every year since 1900, with the exception of 1918, which was the year of the influenza pandemic. Even if cancer becomes the primary cause of mortality, most of what is known concerning lifestyle and dietary change for CVD prevention directly applies to cancer prevention.[4] For example, one of the most dramatic reductions in mortality in US history for CVD and cancer was through a common behavioral/lifestyle change (smoking cessation) that had a profound simultaneous impact on the rates of both diseases. Heart-healthy changes contribute to overall men's health improvements regardless of the part of the human anatomy that is receiving attention, including the penis and the prostate. Heart-healthy changes need to be advocated in urology clinics because this places probability and the research into perspective. Triaging preventive medicine for men's health is providing probability-based advice via evidence-based medicine.

The largest and most recent US and worldwide pharmaceutical-based cancer primary prevention trials that included only men exemplify the immediate need for a more proper perspective. For example, results of the Prostate Cancer Prevention Trial (PCPT) have garnered attention and controversy regarding the use of finasteride daily versus placebo to reduce the risk of prostate cancer.[5–8] The debate about the advantages and disadvantages of finasteride will continue, but a paramount observation from this important trial has not received adequate exposure in the medical literature. More than 18,000 men were included in this randomized trial, and 5 men died of prostate cancer in the finasteride arm and 5 men died of prostate cancer in the placebo arm, but 1123 men in total died during this primary prevention trial.[5] Thus, prostate cancer was responsible for less than 1% of the deaths, whereas most of the mortality was from CVD and other causes. Thus, the results of the first large-scale

[a] Department of Urology, University of Michigan Medical Center, 1500 East Medical Center Drive, Ann Arbor, MI, USA
[b] Eisenhower Wellness Institute, Eisenhower Medical Center, Rancho Mirage, CA, USA
* Department of Urology, University of Michigan Medical Center, 1500 East Medical Center Drive, Ann Arbor, MI.
E-mail address: moyad@umich.edu

Urol Clin N Am 39 (2012) 89–107
doi:10.1016/j.ucl.2011.09.006
0094-0143/12/$ – see front matter © 2012 Published by Elsevier Inc.

men's health PCPT showed that another disease is the primary cause of death in men, and randomized trials accurately reflect day-to-day morbidity and mortality in this regard. This finding does not reduce the seriousness or impact of prostate cancer prevention using a prostate-specific chemoprevention agent, but it places the overall risk of morbidity and mortality in a more proper perspective. Men inquiring about the advantages and disadvantages of finasteride for prostate cancer prevention need to be reminded that the number 1 risk to them in general is CVD, and then the potential prostate cancer risk–specific or men's health consult should occur after this first, more relevant point is discussed, emphasized, and reiterated.

The largest male health dietary supplement clinical trial to prevent cancer was the Selenium and Vitamin E Supplementation Randomized Trial (SELECT).[9] It was terminated approximately 7 years early because of a lack of efficacy, and even a potential negative impact with these high-dose supplements. However, this trial represented a pertinent teaching moment for men's health that once again was missed because of the focus on specific rather than wider issues. SELECT was the largest randomized primary prevention trial of men in urologic and medical history, and once again CVD represented the primary cause of mortality in this study with more than 500 deaths occurring from this cause compared with 1 death from prostate cancer in just 5 years follow-up. Heart-healthy programs need to receive more emphasis in urology and men's health.

The lifestyle recommendations in this article affect CVD and men's health simultaneously. Men can now be offered lifestyle changes that can potentially affect all-cause morbidity and mortality rather than just disease-specific morbidity and mortality.

OPTIMAL MEN'S HEALTH DIET RECOMMENDATION 1

There should be a focus on probability-based changes before focusing on diet, which means that men should know their fasting lipid profile, blood pressure, and other cardiovascular markers as well as they know any other health numerical values, for example prostate-specific antigen (PSA).

The lack of general health knowledge shown by some patients despite an impressive and obsessive need-to-know position concerning prostate, erectile dysfunction (ED), or other health issues is concerning. For example, surveys of the general population indicate that most men do not know their cholesterol values or have little understanding of what they represent in terms of potential health outcomes, and this finding is consistent regardless of age, race, and even gender.[10,11] When the dual concern of CVD and overall men's health risks is emphasized and promoted, men tend to become familiar with all of their clinical values, numbers, and overall risks. For example, it is more relevant to conduct a cholesterol/blood pressure screening and ED or prostate screening on the same day at any institution. Men should also be educated regularly on the normal values of a cholesterol panel and blood pressure test, because these values have recently been updated on 2 different occasions by the Expert Panel from the National Cholesterol Education Program (NCEP).[12,13] A man attending a free PSA screening is at risk of ending up with a myopic health and disease perspective. Preliminary empirical evidence of this concern lies in recent data from Surveillance, Epidemiology and End Results (SEER) tumor registry, which suggests that men diagnosed or treated for prostate cancer need to focus as much on cardiovascular prevention because of the observed competing causes of mortality.[14] At our institution, we have attempted to change our previous paradigm by currently abandoning PSA screening day and organizing, at the least, an annual general health lecture for men. Men need other resources, apart from overburdened primary care doctors, to emphasize and review basic optimal lipid and general health values.[12,13] **Table 1** is a modified, quick review for men and urologic health professionals.

The NCEP suggests a first cholesterol screen at an age of 20 years,[12] which is approximately 20 to 30 years before a suggested PSA test, but few if any men have had a lipid test at this early age. Perhaps clinicians can greatly assist men in adhering to this early screening age. For example, when men with a family history of prostate cancer or ED, or an early diagnosis of most diseases, inquire about what their children should do first to prevent this condition from happening to them, a common suggestion for children or adolescents to just have an initial cholesterol screen seems most appropriate. In my experience, this tends to surprise and simplify patient concerns because most did not previously consider this thought or option for their children. The time is appropriate for this approach because of the recent concern in abnormal lipid levels among adolescents screened in the United States, which is approximately 20% to 43% based on a variety of factors, especially weight status (normal, overweight, or obese).[15]

Table 1
A partial summary of men's health goals for total cholesterol, low-density lipoprotein (LDL), high-density lipoprotein (HDL), and triglyceride with some added modifications that can be used in a clinical setting

Blood Test Parameter	Measurement Commentary
Total cholesterol (mg/dL)	A lower number is better
<160	Optimal
<200	Desirable
200–239	Borderline high
≥240	High
LDL = bad cholesterol (mg/dL)	A lower number is better
<70	Optimal for some high-risk individuals[a]
<100	Optimal
100–129	Near optimal
130–159	Borderline high
160–189	High
≥190	Very high
HDL = good cholesterol (mg/dL)	A higher number is better
<40	Low
40–59	Normal
≥60	High (optimal)
Triglyceride (mg/dL)	A lower number is better
<150	Normal
150–199	Borderline high
200–499	High
≥500	High

[a] High-risk individuals (existing CVD disease or a previous CVD event) may be required to reduce their LDL to less than 70 mg/dL based on new information provided to the Expert Panel.

Data from The Expert Panel. Executive summary of the Third Report of the National Cholesterol Education Program (NCEP). Expert Panel on Detection, Evaluation, and Treatment of High Blood Cholesterol in Adults (Adult Treatment Panel III). JAMA 2001;285:2486–98; and Grundy SM, Cleeman JI, Marz NB, et al. Implications of recent clinical trials for the National Cholesterol Education Program Adult Treatment Panel III Guidelines. Circulation 2004;110:227–39.

CVD risk is affected by lifestyle risk factors such as obesity, physical inactivity, and a high-caloric and overall unhealthy diet. These and other emerging risk factors or risk markers should ideally be discussed, because, despite the cholesterol test being a good marker for predicting future cardiovascular problems, it is not a perfect test. Other novel cardiovascular markers such as high-sensitivity C-reactive protein (hs-CRP), or traditional markers such as impaired fasting glucose or hemoglobin A1c, and evidence of subclinical atherosclerotic disease should also be discussed with the patient.[12,16,17] Even a referral to a cardiologist may be appropriate for some men because some of these markers may also be related to overall mortality as well as CVD risk and some specific men's health conditions.[18]

Additional tangible advantages may occur for a man and his clinician that continue to follow these overall cardiovascular markers. For example, cholesterol levels are an outstanding indicator of how well a patient may be adopting lifestyle changes or even medication compliance following a PSA test, ED diagnosis, or after some definitive therapy. If these numbers improve, it may be more likely that the patient is following a men's health lifestyle program. High-density lipoprotein (HDL) provides a good indicator of the commitment to exercise by the patient. HDL tends to increase, and at times substantially, with a greater amount of aerobic physical activity,[19] and a higher HDL may be correlated with a lower risk of abnormal prostate conditions.[20] Triglycerides are an indicator of changes in belly (visceral) fat, because this compound is generally stored in this anatomic location with increasing blood levels. However, in a minority of patients who follow a healthy lifestyle, a less-than-optimal change in lipid values may occur, but these men can be referred to a specialist for potential drug intervention and more aggressive lifestyle therapy.

Blood pressure monitoring should be emphasized as much as any other values. The Joint National Committee on Prevention, Detection, Evaluation, and Treatment of High Blood Pressure altered the criteria for what defines a healthy blood pressure.[21] Men and their partners should be informed that normal blood pressure is less than 120/80 mm Hg and individuals with a systolic blood pressure of 120 to 139 mm Hg or diastolic blood pressure of 80 to 89 mm Hg are considered to be prehypertensive, and lifestyle changes should be advocated in these individuals (**Table 2**).

Blood pressure can be reduced with a healthier lifestyle,[22] and again is a good indicator of lifestyle compliance, and a healthy blood pressure may also lower the risk of ED.[23] Again, a minority of patients may not reduce their blood pressure with lifestyle changes, but these men can be referred to a specialist. Men who adopt healthy lifestyle and behavioral changes that do not result in CVD risk improvements should still be given encouragement to continue these changes because of the other potentially profound impacts these behaviors may have on overall and mental health.[24,25] Patients seem more motivated to continue healthy lifestyle changes when there is some tangible healthy outcome with the behavioral change, and this becomes more probable when all numbers are used in the consult, including cholesterol and blood pressure, for example, as opposed to just other single and disease-specific (eg, PSA) values.

OPTIMAL MEN'S HEALTH DIET RECOMMENDATION 2

The body mass index (BMI), but more importantly the waist/hip ratio (WHR) or waist circumference (WC) measurement and pant size should also become a standard part of a clinical record before initiating dietary changes.

The negative impact of being overweight or obese on overall morbidity and mortality is well known. BMI is moderately reliable as an isolated measurement, but it is a rapid method to determine who may be overweight or obese.[26] BMI is defined as the weight (in kilograms) divided by the square of the height in meters (kilograms per square meter). Another method to calculate the BMI is to take weight in pounds and divide it by the height in inches squared and to multiply this number by 704 (pounds/inches^2 × 704). A BMI of less than 25 kg/m^2 is considered normal by the Word Health Organization (WHO), whereas 25 to 29 kg/m^2 is overweight, 30 kg/m^2 or more is defined as obese, and 35 kg/m^2 or more is considered morbidly obese. Several of the largest and most recent preventive medicine randomized trials of men or women have shown that most individuals in these studies are overweight at baseline,[5,9,27] and this includes trials to prevent specific men's health abnormalities with prescriptions, supplements, or just dietary change.[5,9,28] Thus, it has become so common to be overweight or obese that only a minority of men in current and past clinical trials have a BMI in the healthy range.

WHR may be another rapid measurement to determine obesity.[26] An individual must stand during the measurement of WHR. WHR more precisely measures abdominal adipose circumference or tissue and fat distribution. The waist is defined as the abdominal circumference midway between the costal margin and the iliac crest. The hip is defined as the largest circumference just below the iliac crest. For men, a WHR greater than 0.90 is a moderate indicator of an increased risk for obesity-related conditions independent of BMI.

WC is perhaps the easiest and fastest method to currently assess obesity, and is my preference, together with pant size (waist size) in men because

Table 2	
A partial summary of the new blood pressure guidelines according to the Joint National Committee on Prevention, Detection, Evaluation, and Treatment of High Blood Pressure	
Systolic/Diastolic Blood Pressure (mm Hg)	**What Does this Mean to Patients?**
Less than 120/80	Normal = low risk
120–139/80–89	Prehypertensive (moderately high or prehigh blood pressure) = moderate risk
140/90 or greater	Hypertensive (high blood pressure) = high risk

Data from Chobanian AV, Bakris GL, Black HR, et al. for the Joint National Committee on Prevention, Detection, Evaluation, and Treatment of High Blood Pressure. National Heart, Lung, and Blood Institute; National High Blood Pressure Education Program Coordinating Committee. Hypertension 2003;42:1206–52.

belly fat (visceral adipose tissue) seems to have one of the best predictive values of CVD and potential all-cause mortality risk among all the other weight measurements from some of the largest prospective studies in the world.[29,30] However, the combination of WC with a BMI measurement may have added predictability. WC is also one of the best predictors of a future cardiovascular event, regardless of the ethnic group studied.[31] WC is also one of the 5 specific criteria of the metabolic syndrome. WC has a tangible advantage compared with BMI, which can be appreciated after an individual commits to resistance exercise. An increase in muscle mass from resistance activities such as weight lifting can cause an increase in BMI, which could be frustrating to the patient and clinician.[26] However, this does not occur when using the WHR or WC measurement. Informing patients of their official WC and asking pant size allows these parameters to not only be documented in the chart but allows for the patient to identify a goal of maintaining or reducing these numbers by the time of the subsequent clinical visit, thereby reducing the emphasis on the weight scale or trying to compete with a national standard. A patient with a BMI of 35 kg/m^2 and a WC of 102 cm may be considered alarming, but a lack of aerobic fitness and caloric restriction, or not being able to reduce the value slightly over time, is more of an issue. A summary of the basic interpretation of the BMI and WC value is presented in **Table 3**.[26]

Kidney stones and renal cell carcinoma (RCC) may have a strong relationship with obesity.[32,33] Obesity is also associated with lower testosterone levels, higher estrogen levels, and a higher risk of CVD, which could partially explain the preliminary finding that obese men have a higher risk of ED,[34–36] but recent novel clinical research suggests that an improvement in these parameters occurs rapidly with just a 10% weight loss from dietary changes alone.[37]

Clinicians should begin to carry and use tape measures that can measure WC, and I often argue that this is as critical as the stethoscope to the individual working in men's health. Clinicians should also refer patients on a consistent basis to ancillary diverse services such as nutritionists, therapists, social workers, a variety of professional and even surgical weight-loss programs if needed, and recent weight-loss consumer publications. Simply becoming familiar with local weight-loss resources is an initial step in the appropriate direction for the patient and clinician.

OPTIMAL MEN'S HEALTH DIET RECOMMENDATION 3

Fitness and overall health should receive more attention. Approximately 30 to 60 minutes or more of physical activity a day on average should be the goal, which should include lifting weights or performing resistance exercises several times a week. Equal emphasis should be placed on aerobic and resistance exercise; one is not more important than the other for men's health.

Physical activity, defined as at least 3 hours of vigorous exercise weekly, was associated with an approximate 70% lower risk of aggressive prostate cancer, advanced disease, and a potential for improved survival in the Health Professionals Follow-up Study.[38] More than 47,000 men were included in this cohort, with a mean follow-up period of 14 years. The investigators appropriately concluded their publication by recommending 30 minutes a day of physical activity for all individuals because of the overall health benefits of this intervention.

Morbidity and mortality from CVD are affected by exercise, but weight lifting also seems to provide additional benefits. For example, additional data were derived from the Health Professionals' Follow-up Study, which prospectively followed more than 44,000 men for 12 years.[39] Men who jogged for 1 hour or more per week had a 42% reduction (*P*<.001 for trend) in the risk of coronary heart disease (CHD), and those who just walked for 30 minutes or more per day or who were involved in other physical activities also experienced a risk reduction in CHD versus

Table 3 BMI and WC values for men's health discussions	
Parameter	**Classification**
BMI	
Less than 25 kg/m^2	Normal weight
25–29 kg/m^2	Overweight
30 kg/m^2 or more	Obese
WC	
Less than 89 cm (35 in) in men	Normal
89–100 cm (35–39 in) in men	Overweight
≥101 cm (≥40 in) in men	Obese

Data from Moyad MA. Current methods used for defining, measuring, and treating obesity. Semin Urol Oncol 2001;19:247–56.

those who did not engage in these activities. Men performing regular resistance exercise (weight lifting) for just 30 minutes or more per week experienced a 23% risk reduction ($P = .03$ for trend) in CHD. This observation was novel because previous prospective studies had not adequately addressed this subject. Weight training can increase fat-free mass and lean body weight, reduce sarcopenia, increase resting metabolic rate, and potentially reduce the risk of abdominal adipose deposition.[40,41] Weight training or resistance training also seems to improve glucose parameters, including insulin sensitivity, and may slightly improve lipid levels, and reduce hypertension,[41,42] which are all potential risk factors for ED and other men's health conditions. Physical activity may also greatly reduce the impact of sympathetic overload that may be one of the many causes of benign prostatic hyperplasia (BPH).[43] These studies emphasize the need to engage in aerobic and resistance activity together because of the documented synergism.

The mental health improvements with increased physical activity seem to be as profound as the physical health benefits.[44,45] For example, a landmark trial was published more than a decade ago that included 156 adult volunteers with major depressive disorder (MDD) randomly assigned a 4-month course of aerobic exercise (30 minutes 3 times/wk), sertraline therapy, or a combination of exercise and sertraline.[46,47] After 4 months, patients in all 3 groups showed significant mental health improvements; however, after 10 months, individuals in the exercise group had significantly lower recurrence rates compared with individuals in the medication arm of the study. Exercising during the follow-up period was associated with a 51% reduction in the risk of a diagnosis of depression at the end of the investigation. Men need to be instructed that regular physical activity and resistance training have adequate physical and mental health benefits such that not performing these activities reduces the potential for improved overall health. It is important to explain to male patients that, if the overall results from exercise studies were viewed similarly to a specific pharmacologic intervention, it probably would have already garnered attention worthy of a Nobel prize in, arguably, multiple categories of medicine, including male health breakthroughs.

OPTIMAL MEN'S HEALTH DIET RECOMMENDATION 4

Men should reduce unhealthy dietary fat intake and increase the consumption of healthy fats, which should lower overall caloric intake. Saturated, trans-fat and even dietary cholesterol should be reduced and replaced by more healthy types of monounsaturated or polyunsaturated fat (eg, ω-3 fatty acids).

Saturated fat reduces low-density lipoprotein (LDL) receptor expression and increases LDL serum levels.[12] LDL increases by 2% for every 1% increase in total calories from saturated fat. The NCEP recommends that saturated fat be reduced to less than 7% of total calories to reduce the risk of CVD. Some nonlean meats, high-fat dairy products (whole milk, butter, cheese, ice cream, and cream), tropical oils (palm oil, coconut oil, and palm kernel oil), baked products and mixed dishes with dairy fats, and shortenings are some of the larger contributors of saturated fat to the food supply. Many foods that contain high levels of saturated fat also contain the highest levels of trans-fat (partially hydrogenated fat), cholesterol, and, more importantly, total calories in many cases. For example, there are almost twice as many calories in 237 mL of whole milk (5 g of saturated fat) compared with skim, or even almond milk or soymilk (0 g of saturated fat each).[48] Thus, identifying 2 similar products, such as milk, meats, dairy, or chips, and choosing the item lower in saturated fat can allow for a profound reduction in total caloric intake, which is critical to helping maintain or reach an appropriate weight or waist size.

However, simply reducing all saturated fat in an individual's diet is not necessarily a practical and healthy dietary lifestyle change. The current cardiovascular goal of obtaining less than 7% of calories from saturated fat seems ideal from past studies, because getting minimal to no calories from saturated fat not only is excessive, it seems to reduce levels of HDL (good cholesterol) from past CVD and men's health clinical trials.[49,50] Reducing almost all saturated fat consumption also suggests that this type of fat, in itself, is heart unhealthy, which is not accurate from the largest recent meta-analysis of prospective studies.[51] In some countries where overall caloric intake is low compared with the United States, saturated fat may have tangible cardiovascular benefits, but this also needs to be placed in perspective.[52] Regions of the world (for example Japan) where healthy men have the largest intakes of saturated fat would still be in the lowest saturated fat consumption category in the United States.[52] Regardless, a potential impact of reducing saturated fat is that it may reduce overall caloric intake and reduce weight and waist gains. Another benefit of reducing saturated fat is that it allows for the opportunity to reduce dietary cholesterol intake and increase the consumption of other monounsaturated and polyunsaturated fats that have shown a greater reduction in CVD from past clinical trials.[53] A summary of the different types of dietary fat, food sources, and impacts on specific lipids is found in **Table 4**.[48]

OPTIMAL MEN'S HEALTH DIET RECOMMENDATION 5

Men should consume a diversity of low-cost fruits, and especially vegetables, and not focus on high-caloric, high-cost, and high-antioxidant exotic juices. Dietary supplements that claim to substitute for fruit and vegetable consumption are also concerning.

Lycopene seemed synonymous with men's health in a variety of media and commercial sources. Few topics in men's health disease prevention enjoyed such excessive attention as lycopene, tomato products, and their potential benefits. For example, an often-cited analysis of more than 80 epidemiologic studies on tomatoes and health seemed to be used by many commercial companies.[54] Approximately half of the studies in this analysis supported the consumption of tomato products at least once a day to reduce the risk of a variety of cancers, including prostate cancer, but a large number of studies in this same analysis failed to detect a correlation. The overall recommendation of the author of the meta-analysis was to increase the consumption of a diversity of

fruits and vegetables and not just tomato products, which was the most critical finding of the analysis that never garnered any commercial attention.

Perception does not seem to reflect reality in this area of nutritional medicine. For example, tomatoes were never the only, or even the primary, source of lycopene. A variety of other healthy products contain this compound, such as apricots, guava, and pink grapefruit.[55] Watermelon is also an adequate source of lycopene, and is the largest source per gram compared with any other source, including tomato products.[56]

Fruits, and especially vegetables in general, have been associated with a reduced risk of some male urologic conditions.[57] For example, the *Brassica* vegetable group is diverse and includes broccoli, Brussels sprouts, cabbage, cauliflower, kale, and watercress, and may slightly reduce the risk of urologic disease,[58] and it is interesting that these products are low in overall calories. The *Allium* vegetables have also been associated with a reduced risk, and this group includes chives, garlic, leeks, onions, and scallions.[59] Fruits and vegetables have unique and shared anticancer and anti–heart disease compounds that may contribute to improved overall health.[57] The sum of the epidemiologic data continues to support the increased consumption of a diversity of fruits and vegetables to potentially and favorably affect men's health, but the overall data currently support a slightly greater potential reduction in CVD risk and mortality,[60] perhaps through assisting in weight loss. Clinicians should

Table 4
Types of dietary fat, some of their primary sources, and the impact on lipid levels and heart health

Type of Dietary Fat	Commonly Found?	Good or Bad Fat, and Impacts on Lipids vs Carbohydrates (Sugars)
Monounsaturated fat (includes ω-9)	Healthy cooking oils (canola, olive, safflower, ...), nuts, ...	Good Lowers LDL Increases HDL
Polyunsaturated fat (includes ω-3 fatty acids)	Healthy cooking oils (canola, soybean, ...), flaxseed, fish, nuts, soybeans, ...	Good Lowers LDL Increases HDL
Saturated fat (also known as hydrogenated fat)	Nonlean meat, high-fat dairy, some fast food	Mostly bad (because it is associated with high caloric intake) Increases LDL Increases HDL
Trans-fat (also known as partially hydrogenated fat)	Some margarine, fast food, snack foods, deep fried foods, ...	Bad Increases LDL Lowers HDL

Data from Moyad MA. Dr Moyad's no bogus science health advice. Ann Arbor (MI): Ann Arbor Media Group; 2009.

recommend fruit and vegetable consumption for better overall health, but not for cancer prevention where the recent large-scale data seems to be less impressive.[61]

Media attention seems to shift from one fruit or vegetable to another with each passing year. Clinicians need to be objective and explain to patients that these media reports do not necessarily represent any major breakthrough, but support the ongoing and past research that consuming a diversity of low-cost fruits and vegetables is just 1 practical and logical approach to improving men's health. A recent example of this controversy is the recent research into pomegranate juice.[62,63] The first attention-gathering study did not include a placebo group or another group of men that consumed another type of healthy juice product.[62] This should not be construed as a lack of efficacy and some of these companies should be lauded for at least investing in research, but an objective overview of the preliminary research and the caloric contribution of these and other juices is necessary. Many brands of pomegranate and other novel juices contain at least 140 calories per 237-mL serving, which translates into more, or at least similar, calories than most commercial regular soft drinks and alcoholic drinks (approximately 100–150 calories).[48,64] Many of these juices are expensive in comparison with cheaper nutritious and lower-calorie products, and it is concerning that low-income patients may find it difficult to afford them. In addition, drug and juice interactions are still being researched, which is important because grapefruit juice studies have provided a paradigm of medication interactions, but novel juices such as pomegranate may also cause some legitimate concerns with medications metabolized by CYP3A4.[65,66]

In partial defense of some of these companies, it is also laudable that some lower-caloric exotic juice options now are appearing on some store shelves.

The competitive nature of the food and beverage industry, like any commercial business, translates into millions of dollars spent yearly on advertising, which usually affects how patients eat and drink. Clinicians need to be advocates for general evidence-based advice instead of encouraging hype on a specific compound or product that does not have at least a moderate amount of evidence in an area of medical need. When a patient begins to depend on a pill alone instead of on a lifestyle change, the potential for seeking other nonlifestyle changes via pills increases.[48] This pendulum of health swings in a bidirectional fashion so, when a patient begins to exercise, there is an increased potential to seek other healthy behavioral changes such as eating better or quitting smoking or consuming less alcohol and not depending on pills. Thus, if a pill count can be kept to a minimum or nonexistent it is rewarding to watch patients depend on lifestyle change as the initial method to correct or prevent a condition. The next recommendation for men in this article would be difficult to achieve with any pill that claims to substitute for a fruit or vegetable; one healthy change improves the likelihood of another healthy lifestyle change.

OPTIMAL MEN'S HEALTH DIET RECOMMENDATION 6

Consume more total (soluble and insoluble) dietary fiber (20–30 g/d) from food for overall health advantages, especially soluble and insoluble fiber, which can easily be found in higher quantities in low-cost options and not just from overcommercialized pills and powders.

General and numerous health benefits from consuming dietary fiber have been well documented and especially include a reduction in CHD risk.[67,68] A pooled analysis of past cohort studies of dietary fiber for the reduction of CHD included research from 10 international studies, which included the United States.[69] In a period of 6 to 10 years of follow-up, and after multivariate adjustment for demographics, BMI, and behavioral changes, each 10 g/d increase of calorie-adjusted total dietary fiber was correlated with a 14% reduction in the risk of total coronary events and a 27% reduction in risk of coronary death. These findings were similar for both genders, and the inverse associations occurred for both soluble (viscous) and insoluble fiber. Past studies have not observed a consistent benefit with one class of fiber rather than the other.[70,71]

Small additions of fiber can affect medication dosages in a positive manner. Only 15 g of psyllium husk supplementation daily with a 10 mg statin (simvastatin) was shown to be as effective as 20 mg of this statin by itself in reducing cholesterol in a preliminary placebo-controlled study of 68 patients over 12 weeks[72] Other cardiovascular benefits have also been consistently found. A meta-analysis of 24 randomized placebo-controlled trials of fiber supplementation found a consistent impact on blood pressure reduction.[73] Supplementation with a mean dose of only 11.5 g/d of fiber reduced systolic blood pressure by 1.13 mm Hg and diastolic pressure by 1.26 mm Hg. The reductions were greater in individuals older than 40 years of age and in hypertensive individuals compared with younger and normotensive participants. Daily intakes of fiber in the United States and many other Western countries is approximately 10 to 15 g/d, which is approximately half of the total amount consistently recommended by the American Heart Association (AHA) and American Dietetic Association (25–30 g/d) for adequate overall health.[74]

Dietary fiber from food is easily achieved from low-cost sources of soluble and insoluble fiber. For example, I often tell patients to have just a third of a cup of a bran cereal, which is only the size of 2 liquor shot glasses, with flaxseed and some fruit, and before they leave home in the morning approximately 20 g of fiber will have already been ingested toward the goal of 25 to 30 g.[48] Low-cost fiber sources such as flaxseed can potentially provide numerous heart-healthy and general men's health benefits and outcomes.[75–79] Flaxseed is also one of the richest plant sources of heart-healthy ω-3 fatty acids, and chia seed is arguably the richest plant source of fiber and ω-3, and both of these additions to the male health diet would be ideal.[48]

However, fiber seems to have become commercialized, and some men are turning primarily toward powders and pills to solve their fiber deficit; this is not only costly, but it also provides primarily small amounts of mostly soluble fiber that make it difficult to reach their total fiber goal using only these sources. For example, I often ask students how many fiber capsules/pills are needed to be consumed daily to obtain just 20 g of fiber, and the answer always seems to provide adequate surprise value (the answer is 30–40 pills a day, depending on the commercial source).[48] Again, research continues to support the overall and heart-healthy benefits of fiber, especially when it is primarily derived from food sources.[80] Arguably, fiber should be advertised to male patients as the ideal internal antiaging product because it lowers blood cholesterol, blood pressure, and reduces the risk of constipation, diverticulitis, hemorrhoids, reflux, and weight gain, which are all conditions associated with aging.

OPTIMAL MEN'S HEALTH DIET RECOMMENDATION 7

Consume moderate (approximately 2 servings or more) weekly intakes of a variety of canned, broiled, baked, and even raw/smoked fatty fish, but fried and high mercury-concentrated fish should be generally discouraged. Other healthy plant-based sources of ω-3 fatty acids (eg, nuts and healthy plant cooking oils) should also be emphasized and consumed. Fish oil

supplements may provide some diverse benefits in moderation.

Ground flaxseed, chia seeds, and soy are good sources of plant-based ω-3 fatty acids (containing α-linolenic acid [ALA]), but numerous types of oily fatty fish also contain high concentrations of marine-based ω-3 fatty acids (eicosapentaenoic acid [EPA] and docosahexaenoic acid [DHA]). Fish are also the best natural food source of vitamin D3 (cholecalciferol), and they contain high concentrations of high-quality protein and minerals.[48] ω-3 Fatty acids have numerous benefits in reducing the risk of a variety of prevalent chronic diseases,[81] especially CVD.[82,83] Potential positive mechanisms of action for fish and fish oil include a reduction in triglycerides,[84] blood pressure,[85] platelet aggregation,[86] and arrhythmias.[87] However, their primary benefit has been their potential ability to reduce the risk of sudden cardiac death (SCD).[88–90] The overall probability of improving some aspect of preventive health when consuming these compounds is noteworthy.[91,92]

A variety of fatty/oily fish contain high levels of ω-3 fatty acids, vitamin D, and protein, including salmon, tuna, sardines, and a variety of other baked, broiled, raw, but not fried, fish are potentially beneficial.[48] Diversity should be encouraged to increase compliance and exposure to a range of nutrients. Research into the benefits of fish consumption to reduce the risk of certain male-specific diseases is in the preliminary stages,[93,94] but a recent meta-analysis suggested that the sum of the evidence points more toward a reduction in prostate cancer mortality compared with morbidity, which is encouraging and should be discussed with patients.[95] However, the role of ω-3 in reducing a cardiovascular event or affecting all-cause mortality is a more definitive conclusion from clinical trials of fish or fish oil consumption for individuals with, and potentially without, a history of heart disease.[96–99]

Average mercury levels in fish have been reported by the US Food and Drug Administration (FDA), but the preliminary data remain controversial and it is not known what clinical impact mercury may have on an individual.[100,101] Four types of larger predatory fish have been most concerning (king mackerel, shark, swordfish, and tilefish) because they have the ability to concentrate larger amounts of methyl-mercury. However, moderate and recommended consumption (2–3 times/wk) of most fish should have minimal impact on human mercury serum levels. A large investigation of moderate mercury serum levels in older individuals found little to no negative long-term impacts on neurobehavioral parameters.[102] A randomized trial of mercury exposure from dental amalgam in children also found no significant health issues.[103] The positive impact of consuming fish seems to outweigh the negative impact in most individuals, with the exception of women considering pregnancy or who are pregnant. Low-cost fish such as anchovies and sardines are low in mercury and have some of the highest concentrations of ω-3 oils that are used in ω-3 fatty acid clinical trials using supplements for heart disease and cancer. In addition, the AHA recommends about 2 servings of fish per week (equivalent to 1 fish oil supplement a day) and plant ω-3 consumption,[104] which I try to reiterate often to urologic patients. Thus, the healthiest sources of ω-3 compounds in food are coincidentally low in mercury.

Tree nuts share some similar clinical positive impacts with marine ω-3 oils. A consistent reduction in the risk of CHD and/or SCD has been associated with an increased consumption of a diversity of nuts in prospective studies, and nuts can also reduce inflammatory markers that affect a variety of organ systems.[105–112] Nuts contain a variety of potential beneficial compounds such as ALA (the primary plant-based ω-3 fatty acid), other polyunsaturated fats, monounsaturated fats, vitamin E, magnesium, potassium, fiber, and flavonoids.[105] However, the primary limitation of tree nuts is their high caloric content, which limits the recommended number of servings per day.

Healthy plant oils used for cooking, such as soybean, canola, olive oil, and safflower, also contain a high concentration of ω-3 fatty acids, monounsaturated fat, and numerous other vitamins and minerals such as natural vitamin E.[48] Most cooking oils contain 120 calories per tablespoon; therefore, moderation again is the cornerstone to good health and nutrition. An extensive review of healthy ω-3 fatty acids can be found in the literature.[91,92]

Primary prevention prospective studies and trials of fish oil supplements are lacking, except for a few examples such as a 2007 study that suggested a benefit with 1800 mg of EPA fish oil daily from a supplement in addition to statin use, which reduced the composite end point of major coronary events by 18%.[99] Subgroup analysis found a benefit for those with preexisting heart disease with higher blood levels of triglycerides and low HDL, or those with abnormal glucose tolerance. Other indirect benefits was the suggestion of lower rates of daily pain (such as back pain) in the fish oil group, but this group also reported higher rates of gastrointestinal and skin reaction side effects from the supplement. Researchers from a recent dietary prospective study of more than 50,000 participants observed a 30% reduced risk of acute coronary syndrome in men, but not women, during a mean follow-up of 7.6 years.[113] The AHA therefore currently recommends a total of 1000 mg/d of the active ingredients in fish oil (EPA and DHA) in patients who have heart disease, which in general is easier to obtain with a supplement and diet in combination. Patients without heart disease are expected to get at least 500 mg/d, which again can be accomplished by consuming 2 fatty fish meals (eg, anchovies, herring, salmon, sardines) per week, or this would be equivalent to 1 fish oil supplement per day. A reduction in triglycerides of 30% to 50% and an improvement in HDL require a total dosage of 3000 to 4000 mg of EPA and DHA per day, which requires a dietary supplement or prescription.[114] The message that will be missed by clinicians and patients in all of the hype and excitement to consume fish oil is the additional benefit of consuming the plant-based ω-3 fatty acids found in seeds, nuts, and oils. In one of the largest randomized trials of a high dietary source of plant ω-3 in patients with prostate cancer, researchers noted a significant increase in the marine ω-3 levels after consuming flaxseed.[78] Plant ω-3 (ALA) gets converted to marine ω-3 (mostly EPA) by the human body in larger quantities than researchers had realized from past studies, which suggests that diversity of ω-3 sources should be the primary goal for an optimal male health diet.

OPTIMAL MEN'S HEALTH DIET RECOMMENDATION 8

Adhere to heart-healthy lifestyle recommendations (numbers 1–7) because the emerging clinical data suggest that these recommendations precisely reflect the most effective male health prevention advice. It is the sum of what is accomplished in moderation that has the highest probability of affecting male health compared with just 1 or several extreme lifestyle changes.

A unique 2-year randomized trial from Italy of vigorous aerobic exercise and diet to improve ED should receive more clinical attention.[115,116] It should change the way health care professionals treat men with ED. A total of 110 obese men (BMI 36–37 kg/m²; ie, morbidly obese), WHR of 1.01 to 1.02, age 43 years, with ED (ED score 13–14 out of 25 [IIEF]), and without diabetes, high cholesterol, or hypertension were included in this trial. A total of 55 men were included in an aggressive-intervention group that involved caloric restriction and increased physical activity via personalized dietary counseling (Mediterranean-style diet), and regular appointments with a personal trainer. Another group of 55 men were in the control group and were given general educational information about exercise and healthy food choices. After 2 years, the BMI significantly decreased on average from 36.9 to 31.2 kg/m^2 in the intervention group, and serum levels of interleukin-6 and C-reactive protein (higher levels are potential indicators of more vascular inflammation) also decreased significantly. The average physical activity level increased significantly from 48 minutes per week to 195 minutes per week in the intervention group, and the mean erectile function score increased significantly from 13.9 to 17. A total of 17 men in the intervention group reported an erectile score of 22 or higher (normal function). Several changes were independently and significantly associated with a higher rate of improved erections, including a lower BMI or BMI reduction, increased physical activity, and lower C-reactive protein levels. Approximately 33% of the men in this study with ED regained normal erectile function after 2 years of following healthy behaviors primarily from exercise, weight reduction, caloric control, and healthy dietary changes. This clinical trial had 1 major limitation, which was the lack of examining the impact of psychological factors and social intervention, because these lifestyle changes could have improved mood, self-esteem, and reduced depression, and this could have also been a reason for improved erectile function. However, the combined healthy changes in the intervention group that occurred after 2 years were notable and diverse:

- Total caloric reduction of 390 calories/d (from 2340 to 1950 calories)
- Complex carbohydrate increase and simple sugar reduction
- Fiber consumption increased by 10 g a day (from 15 to 25 g)
- Protein consumption increased
- No change in the overall percentage of fat in the diet (30% of calories), but a reduction in saturated fat (from 14% to 9%) and an increased intake in monounsaturated fat (from 9% to 14%)
- Ratios of ω-6 to ω-3 fatty acids was reduced by half (from 12 to 6)
- Cholesterol was reduced from dietary sources by 84 mg/d (from 360 to 276 mg/d)
- Exercise time (mainly walking) increased from about 7 minutes/d to almost 30 minutes/d

- Average weight loss was 15 kg (from 102.8 to 87.8 kg)
- Average BMI decreased by almost 6 points (from 36.9 to 31.2 kg/m^2)
- WHR decreased by 0.09 (from 1.02 to 0.93)
- Erectile function scores increased by 3 points (from 13.9 to 17 points)
- Blood pressure decreased by 3 to 4 points; systolic from 127 to 124 mm Hg, and diastolic from 86 to 82 mm Hg
- Total cholesterol decreased by 11 mg/dL (from 213 to 202 mg/dL), but HDL (good cholesterol) increased by 9 points (from 39 to 48 mg/dL)
- Triglycerides decreased by 19 mg/dL (from 169 to 150 mg/dL)
- Glucose decreased by 8 mg/dL (from 103 to 95 mg/dL) and insulin level also decreased by 7 points (from 21 to 14 μU/mL)
- CRP was reduced by1.4 mg/L (from 3.3 to 1.9 mg/L)
- Interleukin-6 was reduced by 1.4 pg/mL (from 4.5–3.1 pg/mL)
- Interleukin-8 (IL-8, another inflammatory marker) was reduced by 1.2 pg/mL (from 5.3 to 4.1 pg/mL).

Other lifestyle modifications, including tobacco cessation, should be considered to reduce all-cause mortality including cancer,[117–120] and potentially to reduce the risk of specific male health conditions.[121] Moderate alcohol consumption, regardless of the source, also seems to reduce cardiovascular events,[122] and is part of the Mediterranean diet. However, alcohol follows a U-shaped curve, which is why, when consumed in excess, the detriments of alcohol outweigh the benefits.

Past general studies of men have shown that few (less than 5%) have reported adhering to numerous moderate healthy behaviors at one time.[123] Studies of combined moderate lifestyle changes continue to suggest that it is the sum of what is accomplished, rather than 1 or 2 specific behavioral changes, that can affect cardiovascular markers, CVD, cancer, and all-cause mortality.[124] Thus, I often use checklists derived and modified from the Mediterranean diet US study,[125] and the 52-countries study and other combined male lifestyle studies to ensure verve and compliance in patients.[126–130] These studies found that, regardless of race, age, genetics, and geographic location around the world, the ability to maintain numerous consistent features of lifestyle and/or diet was associated with a 85% to 95% reduced risk of a cardiovascular event, and similar behaviors and changes in other recent studies showed

Table 5
US Mediterranean diet study. Individuals with scores of 6 or more on the checklist had a lower risk of early mortality compared with those with scores of 4 or less. Review the checklist, and add up the points

Beverage or Food	Answer Yes or No (1 Point for Each Question Answered Yes and 0 Points for a No)
Alcohol: 2 drinks a day or less for men and 1 drink or less for women	
Fat intake focused on healthy fats, mostly monounsaturated and polyunsaturated (eg, canola, olive, safflower oil)	
Fish: at least 2 or more servings per week	
Fruit: 4 or more servings a day	
Legumes/beans: 2 or more servings a week	
Meat: 1 or less servings a day	
Nuts and seeds: 2 or more servings a week	
Vegetables (other than potatoes): 4 or more servings a day	
Whole grains (eg, whole grain/multigrain and whole wheat foods with large amount of fiber and protein): 2 or more servings a day	
Total score	

Note: Traditional Mediterranean diets also allow moderate intakes of dairy, such as cheese, milk, and yogurt.
Data from Moyad MA. Dr Moyad's no bogus science health advice. Ann Arbor (MI): Ann Arbor Media Group; 2009.

an improved ability to live beyond average life expectancy with minimal mental or physical morbidity. The critical characteristics in these individuals included behavioral changes with no commentary or benefit or detriment in taking a dietary supplement. **Table 5** is a modified checklist that I provide to individuals seeking to increase their odds or probability of living longer and better through dietary changes adapted from a Mediterranean diet.[48] Other checklists can be obtained from 2 other publications that are widely available to the clinician and patient.[48,64] How many men, or even colleagues, have all of these features or need to work on these changes? How many male health conditions could be prevented or improved with these heart-healthy changes?

OPTIMAL MEN'S HEALTH DIET RECOMMENDATION 9

Less is more. Multivitamins and vitamin D have the potential to be overrated and adult men who desire to consume these specific supplements should not take more than 1 children's multivitamin a day or an 800 to 1000 IU vitamin D supplement if found deficient on a reliable blood test.

Despite a lack of rigorous or even minimal scientific evidence, multivitamins are the largest selling and used supplements in the United States.[131] They are also the primary supplement used by men in notable prostate cancer screening studies,[132] male health prevention trials,[133] and by male physicians.[134] Why? Perhaps it is the perception compared with the reality of the evidence, but until some higher quality evidence finds some realistic benefit with these supplements, the potential for harm when taking them in excess is concerning.[135] For example, an increased risk of advanced and fatal prostate was found in one of the largest prospective epidemiologic studies of multivitamins, and the greater use of other supplements was also associated with an even greater risk.[136] Men with a family history of prostate cancer experienced the largest and most significant increased risks of this condition. Other large male observational studies have found similar results.[137,138] Some recent studies in breast cancer have mirrored these negative findings.[139,140] Multivitamins are also replete with higher doses of B vitamins, which have also recently been found to have no impact on health or increase the risk of prostate cancer in the largest and most recent meta-analysis of clinical trials.[141,142] Regardless of the side of the argument that one supports, there is no consistent suggestion of benefit with a greater intake of multivitamins, and because there is a suggestion of either no impact or serious harm, it is prudent to wait for more clarity from more clinical studies.[143]

Some insight was provided in the Supplementation en Vitamines et Mineraux Antioxydants (SUVIMAX) randomized, placebo-controlled trial that included several vitamins and minerals at moderate or low dosages not usually used in clinical trials,[144] and commonly found in children's formulations. SUVIMAX was a randomized, double-blind, placebo-controlled primary prevention trial (participants were healthy at the start of the trial). A total of 13,017 French adults (7876 women aged 35–60 years and 5141 men aged 45–60 years) were included in this study. All of the individuals took either a placebo or a daily capsule that consisted of:

- 120 mg of vitamin C
- 30 mg of vitamin E
- 6 mg of β-carotene
- 100 μg of selenium
- 20 mg of zinc.

These individuals were followed for 7.5 years. Nothing remarkable occurred in the group as a whole, but men experienced a nonsignificant ($P = .54$) 18% reduction in ischemic cardiovascular risk, a significant ($P = .008$) 31% reduction in risk of being diagnosed with cancer, and a significant ($P = .02$) 37% reduction in the risk of dying from any cause. It seemed that taking a low-dose multivitamin minimally based formula could provide a potential benefit for some men. The researchers from this study suggested that men benefited because they had lower levels of these vitamins and minerals in their blood from less-than-optimal dietary patterns at the beginning of the study compared with the women, who consumed a more healthy diet on average. A follow-up secondary observation to this study (8.8–9 years) found that this multivitamin reduced the risk of prostate cancer by 48% in men with a low PSA (less than 3), but in men with a higher PSA, a multivitamin may have been associated with a higher risk of being diagnosed with prostate cancer.[145] Therefore, if a man has an increased PSA, he should be careful about taking dietary supplements to reduce risk. This multivitamin did not affect PSA or insulinlike growth factor levels, suggesting that risk was affected by other methods. Older age (average age of men, 51 years), higher BMI, and men with higher PSA levels also had a significantly increased risk for prostate cancer. Side effects from the low-dose

multivitamin were similar to placebo. One limitation in this study was that no information was collected on family history of prostate cancer. Because this is arguably the best evidence to date for men's health and the consumption of a mixed supplement product, it would be wise not to take anything larger than a children's multivitamin per day until someone can show that more is better, which, as mentioned earlier, is not the case. In SUVIMAX, the ability for this low-dose pill to do harm in men (those with a high PSA) should not be dismissed. Waiting for the results of the first randomized US trial of adult men only (Physicians Health Study II) taking a daily multivitamin should be available soon,[146] and should provide more clarity in this currently nebulous situation.

Vitamin D seems fraught with as many issues as multivitamins. The tendency for patients to ingest more of this supplement is enticing but, in men's health, vitamin D has not been impressive and, in several studies, no impact or potential harm have been shown at higher blood levels.[147] There is little doubt that vitamin D is important for bone health, but in my opinion the amount needed has been embellished and exaggerated. Vitamin D tends to function like a hormone, which is why caution should be exercised because the potential for a U-shaped risk curve exists (similar to alcohol and other hormones) for male health.[148] During the time of submission of this article, one of the largest and longest randomized trials in women found that excessively high blood levels of vitamin D from supplementation compared with placebo was associated with an increased risk of falls and fractures.[149] In my opinion, the normal level of vitamin D should be from 30 to 40 ng/mL based on this study and expert opinion from a review of past clinical trials accessing multiple outcomes.[150] A total of 1000 IU (25 μg) of vitamin D is adequate to increase blood levels of vitamin D over time, and a suggestion of outright deficiency from consistent, reliable blood testing may lead to higher intakes. However, even vitamin D blood tests have a history of uncertainty based on the assay used.[151,152] Monitoring vitamin D in men, especially higher risk patients with bone loss, for example men on luteinizing hormone–releasing hormone medications for prostate cancer may be appropriate,[64] but, in general for men's health, the vitamin D test may provide more harm than good until more clinical endpoints are followed in healthy individuals.[152]

One additional point about vitamin D merits consideration. It could be that vitamin D blood levels are simply a marker of healthy behavior. A young, lean man, with low cholesterol who consumes fish and exercises outside regularly is more likely to have a higher blood level of vitamin D compared with an older, physically inactive obese man with a high cholesterol level.[48] Is it really the vitamin D supplement providing the most benefit for men's health, or the finding that higher vitamin D levels could be found on average in more healthy men?

OPTIMAL MEN'S HEALTH DIET RECOMMENDATION 10

Cholesterol lowering through diet, lifestyle, medications (statins), and supplements is underrated and should potentially be considered to be the real so-called male multivitamin.

Statins should have been given a large clinical trial to prevent male health conditions compared with any dietary supplement or another drug based on the plethora of past evidence.[153–156] It could be argued that it is too difficult to conduct such a trial when a large proportion of men are already taking these medications, but this does not apply when using the JUPITER trial as the most recent example of the great potential impact on cardiovascular health when aggressive lipid lowering is accomplished in individuals who are in no apparent immediate need of such intervention.[157,158] In addition, emerging clinical data continue to support the use of cholesterol lowering as one of best potential methods of reducing the risk of aggressive prostate cancer,[159,160] which arguably makes this intervention the ideal potential male health preventive method. Ongoing research in other areas of men's health also support the use of cholesterol lowering to achieve optimal results.[161,162] Thus, if not cholesterol lowering through diet, exercise, supplements, and perhaps statin use, then what other agent provides a better risk/benefit ratio? Even if aggressive cholesterol lowering were found to be ineffective for specific male health conditions (BPH, ED, prostate cancer), but only reduced the risk of dying younger from all causes,[163] or only reduced the number 1 cause of death in men,[157] then I would be content with this finding.

SUMMARY

Other, simplistic dietary changes could have been proffered in this article, such as sodium reduction and increased amounts of sleep, but these and other changes should be addressed in another publication focused on overall health, regardless of gender.[48,64] In the meantime, why wait for any more recommendations, evidence, or even motivation? Clinicians have access to a wealth of data that suggest that an optimal male diet and overall program does exist to reduce the primary causes of morbidity and mortality in men, and many of these recommendations are outlined in this article. Whether it is incorporating moderation in terms of behavioral changes, or reducing or increasing dietary supplement or medication use, the time to triage men's health is now. Health care professionals must prioritize these changes in all aspects of their behavior and this has not been an easy task. Official treatment guidelines in urology need to focus as much on lifestyle changes and supplements that are, and are not, effective, as on other medical interventions. When this occurs, I believe patients will take our recommendations more seriously but, until that time, articles that continue to advocate an optimal health program may be a step in the right direction.

REFERENCES

1. Lloyd-Jones D, Adams RJ, Brown TM, et al. Heart disease and stroke statistics-2010 update: a report from the American Heart Association. Circulation 2010;121:e46–215.
2. Bonow RO, Smaha LA, Smith SC, et al. The international burden of cardiovascular disease: responding to the emerging epidemic. Circulation 2002;106:1602–5.
3. World Heart Federation web site. Available at: http://www.world-heart-federation.org. Accessed March 20, 2010.
4. Eyre H, Kahn R, Robertson RM, et al. Preventing cancer, cardiovascular disease, and diabetes: a common agenda for the American Cancer Society, the American Diabetes Association, and the American Heart Association. Circulation 2004;109:3244–55.
5. Thompson IM, Goodman PJ, Tangen CM, et al. The influence of finasteride on the development of prostate cancer. N Engl J Med 2003;349:215–24.
6. Scardino PT. The prevention of prostate cancer-the dilemma continues. N Engl J Med 2003;349:297–9.
7. Reynolds T. Prostate cancer prevention trial yields positive results, but with a few cautions. J Natl Cancer Inst 2003;95:1030–1.
8. Kaplan SA, Roehrborn CG, Meehan AG, et al. PCPT: evidence that finasteride reduces risk of most frequently detected intermediate- and high-grade (Gleason score 6 and 7) cancer. Urology 2009;73:935–9.
9. Lippman SM, Klein EA, Goodman PJ, et al. Effect of selenium and vitamin E on risk of prostate cancer and other cancers: the Selenium and Vitamin E Cancer Prevention Trial (SELECT). JAMA 2009;301:39–51.
10. Nash IS, Mosca L, Blumenthal RS, et al. Contemporary awareness and understanding of cholesterol

as a risk factor: results of an American Heart Association National Survey. Arch Intern Med 2003;163: 1597–600.

11. Hickey A, O'Hanlon A, McGee H, et al. Stroke awareness in the general population: knowledge of stroke risk factors and warning signs in older adults. BMC Geriatr 2009;9:35.

12. The Expert Panel. Executive summary of the Third Report of the National Cholesterol Education Program (NCEP). Expert Panel on Detection, Evaluation, and Treatment of High Blood Cholesterol in Adults (Adult Treatment Panel III). JAMA 2001;285: 2486–98.

13. Grundy SM, Cleeman JI, Marz NB, et al. Implications of recent clinical trials for the National Cholesterol Education Program Adult Treatment Panel III Guidelines. Circulation 2004;110:227–39.

14. Ketchandji M, Kuo YF, Shahinian VB, et al. Cause of death in older men after the diagnosis of prostate cancer. J Am Geriatr Soc 2009;57:24–30.

15. Centers for Disease Control and Prevention (CDC). Prevalence of abnormal lipid levels among youths-United States, 1999-2006. MMWR Morb Mortal Wkly Rep 2010;59:29–33.

16. Ridker PM. Clinical application of C-reactive protein for cardiovascular disease detection and prevention. Circulation 2003;107:363–9.

17. Ridker PM, Cannon CP, Morrow D, et al. C-reactive protein levels and outcomes after statin therapy. N Engl J Med 2005;352:20–8.

18. Chang ST, Chu CM, Hsu JT, et al. Independent determinants of coronary artery disease in erectile dysfunction patients. J Sex Med 2010;7(4 Pt 1): 1478–87.

19. Kraus WE, Houmard JA, Duscha BD, et al. Effects of the amount and intensity of exercise on plasma lipoproteins. N Engl J Med 2002;347:1483–92.

20. Hammarsten J, Hogstedt B. Hyperinsulinaemia as a risk factor for developing benign prostatic hyperplasia. Eur Urol 2001;39:151–8.

21. Chobanian AV, Bakris GL, Black HR, et al. Seventh report of the Joint National Committee on Prevention, Detection, Evaluation, and Treatment of High Blood Pressure. Hypertension 2003; 42:1206–52.

22. Whelton SP, Chin A, Xin X, et al. Effect of aerobic exercise on blood pressure: a meta-analysis of randomized, controlled trials. Ann Intern Med 2002;136:493–503.

23. Ponholzer A, Temmi C, Mock K, et al. Prevalence and risk factors for erectile dysfunction in 2869 men using a validated questionnaire. Eur Urol 2005;47:80–5.

24. Strijk JE, Proper KI, Klaver L, et al. Associations between VO_2max and vitality in older workers: a cross-sectional study. BMC Public Health 2010; 10:684.

25. Blair SN, Morris JN. Healthy hearts-and the universal benefits of being physically active: physical activity and health. Ann Epidemiol 2009;19: 253–6.

26. Moyad MA. Current methods used for defining, measuring, and treating obesity. Semin Urol Oncol 2001;19:247–56.

27. Writing Group for the Women's Health Initiative Investigators. Risks and benefits of estrogen plus progestin in healthy postmenopausal women: principal results from the Women's Health Initiative randomized controlled trial. JAMA 2002;288:321–33.

28. Shike M, Latkany L, Riedel E, et al. Lack of effect of a low-fat, high-fruit, -vegetable, and -fiber diet on serum prostate-specific antigen of men without prostate cancer: results from a randomized trial. J Clin Oncol 2002;20:3592–8.

29. Pischon T, Boeing H, Hoffmann K, et al. General and abdominal adiposity and risk of death in Europe. N Engl J Med 2008;359:2105–20.

30. Jacobs EJ, Newton CC, Wang Y, et al. Waist circumference and all-cause mortality in a large US cohort. Arch Intern Med 2010;170:1293–301.

31. Zhu S, Heymsfield SB, Toyoshima H, et al. Race-ethnicity-specific waist circumference cutoffs for identifying cardiovascular disease risk factors. Am J Clin Nutr 2005;81:409–15.

32. Taylor EN, Stampfer MJ, Curhan GC. Obesity, weight gain, and the risk of kidney stones. JAMA 2005;293:455–62.

33. Moyad MA. Obesity, interrelated mechanisms, and exposures and kidney cancer. Semin Urol Oncol 2001;19:270–9.

34. Riedner CE, Rhoden EL, Ribeiro EP, et al. Central obesity is an independent predictor of erectile dysfunction in older men. J Urol 2006;176:1519–23.

35. Bacon CG, Mittleman MA, Kawachi I, et al. Sexual function in men older than 50 years of age: results from the Health Professionals Follow-up Study. Ann Intern Med 2003;139:161–8.

36. Walczak MK, Lokhandwala N, Hodge MB, et al. Prevalence of cardiovascular risk factors in erectile dysfunction. J Gend Specif Med 2002; 5:19–24.

37. Khoo J, Piantadosi C, Worthley S, et al. Effects of low-energy diet on sexual function and lower urinary tract symptoms in obese men. Int J Obes 2010;34:1396–403.

38. Giovannucci EL, Liu Y, Leitzmann MF, et al. A prospective study of physical activity and incident and fatal prostate cancer. Arch Intern Med 2005;165:1005–10.

39. Tanasescu M, Leitzmann MF, Rimm EB, et al. Exercise type and intensity in relation to coronary heart disease in men. JAMA 2002;288:1994–2000.

40. Poehlman ET, Melby C. Resistance training and energy balance. Int J Sport Nutr 1998;8:143–59.

41. Braith RW, Stewart KJ. Resistance exercise training: its role in the prevention of cardiovascular disease. Circulation 2006;113:2642–50.

42. Hurley BF, Roth SM. Strength training in the elderly. Sports Med 2000;30:249–68.

43. Platz EA, Kawachi I, Rimm EB, et al. Physical activity and benign prostatic hyperplasia. Arch Intern Med 1998;158:2349–56.

44. Blake H, Mo P, Malik S, et al. How effective are physical activity interventions for alleviating depressive symptoms in older people? A systematic review. Clin Rehabil 2009;23:873–87.

45. Deslandes A, Moraes H, Ferreira C, et al. Exercise and mental health: many reasons to move. Neuropsychobiology 2009;59:191–8.

46. Blumenthal JA, Babyak MA, Moore KA, et al. Effects of exercise training on older patients with major depression. Arch Intern Med 1999;159:2349–56.

47. Babyak M, Blumenthal JA, Herman S, et al. Exercise treatment for major depression: maintenance of therapeutic benefit at 10 months. Psychosom Med 2000;62:633–8.

48. Moyad MA. Dr Moyad's no bogus science health advice. Ann Arbor (MI): Ann Arbor Media Group; 2009.

49. Yu JN, Cunningham JA, Rosenberg Thouin S, et al. Hyperlipidemia. Prim Care 2000;27:541–87.

50. Ornish D, Weidner G, Fair WR, et al. Intensive lifestyle changes may affect the progression of prostate cancer. J Urol 2005;174:1065–9.

51. Siri-Tarino PW, Sun Q, Hu FB, et al. Meta-analysis of prospective cohort studies evaluating the association of saturated fat with cardiovascular disease. Am J Clin Nutr 2010;91:535–46.

52. Yamagishi K, Iso H, Yatsuya H, et al. Dietary intake of saturated fatty acids and mortality from cardiovascular disease in Japanese: the Japan Collaborative Cohort Study for Evaluation of Cancer Risk (JACC) Study. Am J Clin Nutr 2010;92:759–65.

53. Mozaffarian D, Micha R, Wallace S. Effects of coronary heart disease of increasing polyunsaturated fat in place of saturated fat: a systematic review and meta-analysis of randomized controlled trials. PLoS Med 2010;7:e1000252.

54. Giovannucci E. Tomatoes, tomato-based products, lycopene, and cancer: review of the epidemiologic literature. J Natl Cancer Inst 1999;91:317–31.

55. Moyad MA. The ABCs of nutrition and supplements for prostate cancer. Ann Arbor (MI): JW Edwards Publishers; 2000.

56. Available at: www.usda.gov. Accessed October 25, 2010.

57. Cohen JH, Kristal AR, Stanford JL. Fruit and vegetable intakes and prostate cancer risk. J Natl Cancer Inst 2000;92:61–8.

58. Kristal AR, Lampe JW. Brassica vegetables and prostate cancer risk: a review of the epidemiological evidence. Nutr Cancer 2002;42:1–9.

59. Hsing AW, Chokkalingam AP, Gao YT, et al. Allium vegetables and risk of prostate cancer: a population-based study. J Natl Cancer Inst 2002;94:1648–51.

60. Walker C, Reamy BV. Diets for cardiovascular disease prevention: what is the evidence? Am Fam Physician 2009;79:571–8.

61. Boffetta P, Couto E, Wichmann J, et al. Fruit and vegetable intake and overall cancer risk in the European Prospective Investigation into Cancer and Nutrition (EPIC). J Natl Cancer Inst 2010;102:1–9.

62. Pantuck AJ, Leppert JT, Zomorodian N, et al. Phase II study of pomegranate juice for men with rising prostate-specific antigen following surgery or radiation for prostate cancer. Clin Cancer Res 2006;12(13):4018–26.

63. Forest CP, Padma-Nathan H, Liker HR. Efficacy and safety of pomegranate juice on improvement of erectile dysfunction in male patients with mild to moderate erectile dysfunction: a randomized, placebo-controlled, double-blind, cross-over study. Int J Impot Res 2007;19:564–7.

64. Moyad MA. Promoting wellness for prostate cancer patients. 3rd edition. Ann Arbor (MI): Ann Arbor Media Group; 2010.

65. Uno T, Yasui-Furukori N. Effect of grapefruit juice in relation to human pharmacokinetic study. Curr Clin Pharmacol 2006;1:157–61.

66. Komperda KE. Potential interaction between pomegranate juice and warfarin. Pharmacotherapy 2009;29:1002–6.

67. Van Horn L. Fiber, lipids, and coronary heart disease. Nutrition Committee advisory. Circulation 1997;95:2701–4.

68. Brown L, Rosner B, Willett WW, et al. Cholesterol-lowering effects of dietary fiber: a meta-analysis. Am J Clin Nutr 1999;69:30–42.

69. Pereira MA, O'Reilly E, Augustsson K, et al. Dietary fiber and risk of coronary heart disease: a pooled analysis of cohort studies. Arch Intern Med 2004;164:370–6.

70. Pietinen P, Rimm EB, Korhonen P, et al. Intake of dietary fiber and risk of coronary heart disease in a cohort of Finnish men: the Alpha-Tocopherol, Beta-Carotene Cancer Prevention Study. Circulation 1996;94:2720–7.

71. Rimm EB, Ascherio A, Giovannucci E, et al. Vegetable, fruit, and cereal fiber intake and risk of coronary heart disease among men. JAMA 1996;275:447–51.

72. Moreyra AE, Wilson AC, Koraym A. Effect of combining psyllium fiber with simvastatin in lowering cholesterol. Arch Intern Med 2005;165:1161–6.

73. Streppel MT, Arends LR, van't Veer P, et al. Dietary fiber and blood pressure: a meta-analysis of randomized placebo-controlled trials. Arch Intern Med 2005;165:150–6.

74. Marlett JA, McBurney MI, Slavin JL, et al. Position of the American Dietetic Association: health implications of dietary fiber. J Am Diet Assoc 2002; 102:993–1000.

75. Pan A, Yu D, Demark-Wahnefried W, et al. Meta-analysis of the effects of flaxseed interventions on blood lipids. Am J Clin Nutr 2009;90:288–97.

76. Demark-Wahnefried W, Price DT, Polascik TJ, et al. Pilot study of dietary fat restriction and flaxseed supplementation in men with prostate cancer before surgery: exploring the effects on hormonal levels, prostate-specific antigen, and histopathologic features. Urology 2001;58:47–52.

77. Demark-Wahnefried W, Robertson CN, Walther PJ, et al. Pilot study to explore effects of low-fat, flaxseed-supplemented diet on proliferation of benign prostatic epithelium and prostate-specific antigen. Urology 2004;63:900–4.

78. Demark-Wahnefried W, Polascik TJ, George SL, et al. Flaxseed supplementation (not dietary fat restriction) reduces prostate cancer proliferation rates in men presurgery. Cancer Epidemiol Biomarkers Prev 2008;17:3577–87.

79. Zhang W, Wang X, Liu Y, et al. Effects of dietary flaxseed lignan extract on symptoms of benign prostatic hyperplasia. J Med Food 2008;11:207–14.

80. Anderson JW, Baird P, Davis RH Jr, et al. Health benefits of dietary fiber. Nutr Rev 2009;67:188–205.

81. Morris MC, Evans DA, Bienias JL, et al. Consumption of fish and n-3 fatty acids and risk of incident Alzheimer disease. Arch Neurol 2003;60:940–6.

82. Bucher HC, Hengstler P, Schindler C, et al. N-3 polyunsaturated fatty acids in coronary heart disease: a meta-analysis of randomized controlled trials. Am J Med 2002;112:298–304.

83. Kris-Etherton PM, Harris WS, Appel LJ, et al. Fish consumption, fish oil, omega-3 fatty acids, and cardiovascular disease. Circulation 2002;106:2747–57.

84. Harris WS. N-3 fatty acids and serum lipoproteins: human studies. Am J Clin Nutr 1997;65(Suppl 5): 1645S–54S.

85. Morris MC, Sacks F, Rosner B. Does fish oil lower blood pressure? A meta-analysis of controlled trials. Circulation 1993;88:523–33.

86. Mori TA, Beilin LJ, Burke V, et al. Interactions between dietary fat, fish, and fish oils and their effects on platelet function in men at risk of cardiovascular disease. Arterioscler Thromb Vasc Biol 1997;17:279–86.

87. Christensen JH, Korup E, Aaroe J, et al. Fish consumption, n-3 fatty acids in cell membranes, and heart rate variability in survivors of myocardial infarction with left ventricular dysfunction. Am J Cardiol 1997;79:1670–3.

88. Leaf A, Kang JX, Xiao YF, et al. Clinical prevention of sudden cardiac death by n-3 polyunsaturated fatty acids and mechanism of prevention of arrhythmias by n-3 fish oils. Circulation 2003;107: 2646–52.

89. Albert CM, Campos H, Stampfer MJ, et al. Blood levels of long-chain n-3 fatty acids and the risk of sudden death. N Engl J Med 2002;346:1113–8.

90. Kromhout D. Fish consumption and sudden cardiac death. JAMA 1998;279:65–6.

91. Moyad MA. An introduction to dietary/supplemental omega-3 fatty acids for general health and prevention: Part I. Urol Oncol 2005;23:28–35.

92. Moyad MA. An introduction to dietary/supplemental omega-3 fatty acids for general health and prevention: part II. Urol Oncol 2005;23:36–48.

93. Augustsson K, Michaud DS, Rimm EB, et al. A prospective study of intake of fish and marine fatty acids and prostate cancer. Cancer Epidemiol Biomarkers Prev 2003;12:64–7.

94. Yang YJ, Lee SH, Hong SJ, et al. Comparison of fatty acid profiles in the serum of patients with prostate cancer and benign prostatic hyperplasia. Clin Biochem 1999;32:405–9.

95. Szymanski KM, Wheeler DC, Mucci LA. Fish consumption and prostate cancer risk: a review and meta-analysis. Am J Clin Nutr 2010;92:1223–33.

96. Burr ML, Fehily AM, Gilbert JF, et al. Effects of changes in fat, fish, and fibre intakes on death and myocardial reinfarction: Diet and Reinfarction Trial (DART). Lancet 1989;2:757–61.

97. GISSI-Prevenzione Investigators. Dietary supplementation with n-3 polyunsaturated fatty acids and vitamin E after myocardial infarction: results from the GISSI-Prevenzione trial. Lancet 1999;354:447–55.

98. Marchioli R, Barzi F, Bomba E, et al. Early protection against sudden cardiac death by n-3 polyunsaturated fatty acids after myocardial infarction: time-course analysis of the results of the Gruppo Italiano per lo Studio della Sopravvivenza nell'Infarto Miocardico (GISSI)-Prevenzione. Circulation 2002;105:1897–903.

99. Yokoyama M, Origasa H, Matsuzaki M, et al. Effects of eicosapentaenoic acid on major coronary events in hypercholesterolaemic patients (JELIS): a randomized open-label, blinded endpoint analysis. Lancet 2007;369:1090–8.

100. Guallar E, Sanz-Gallardo MI, van't Veer P, et al. Mercury, fish oils, and the risk of myocardial infarction. N Engl J Med 2002;347:1747–54.

101. Yoshizawa K, Rimm EB, Morris JJ, et al. Mercury and the risk of coronary heart disease in men. N Engl J Med 2002;347:1755–60.

102. Weil M, Bressler J, Parsons P, et al. Blood mercury levels and neurobehavioral function. JAMA 2005; 293:1875–82.

103. DeRouen TA, Martin MD, Leroux BG, et al. Neurobehavioral effects of dental amalgam in children: a randomized clinical trial. JAMA 2006; 295:1784–92.

104. Kris-Etherton PM, Harris WS, Appel LJ, et al. Omega-3 fatty acids and cardiovascular disease: new recommendations from the American Heart Association. Arterioscler Thromb Vasc Biol 2003; 23:151–2.

105. Albert CM, Gaziano JM, Willett WC, et al. Nut consumption and decreased risk of sudden cardiac death in the physicians' health study. Arch Intern Med 2002;162:1382–7.

106. Ellsworth JL, Kushi LH, Folsom AR. Frequent nut intake and risk of death from coronary heart disease and all causes in postmenopausal women: the Iowa Women's Health Study. Nutr Metab Cardiovasc Dis 2001;11:372–7.

107. Hu FB, Willett WC. Optimal diets for prevention of coronary heart disease. JAMA 2002;288:2569–78.

108. Hu FB, Stampfer MJ, Manson JE, et al. Frequent nut consumption and risk of coronary heart disease: prospective cohort study. BMJ 1998;317:1341–5.

109. Fraser GE, Shavlik DJ. Risk factors for all-cause and coronary heart disease mortality in the oldest-old: the Adventist Health Study. Arch Intern Med 1997;157:2249–58.

110. Fraser GE, Sabate J, Beeson WL, et al. A possible protective effect of nut consumption on risk of coronary heart disease: the Adventist Health Study. Arch Intern Med 1992;152:1416–24.

111. Sabate J, Wien M. Nuts, blood lipids and cardiovascular disease. Asia Pac J Clin Nutr 2010;19: 131–6.

112. Casas-Agustench P, Bullo M, Salas-Salvado J. Nuts, inflammation and insulin resistance. Asia Pac J Clin Nutr 2010;19:124–30.

113. Bjerregaard LJ, Joensen AM, Dethlefsen C, et al. Fish intake and acute coronary syndrome. Eur Heart J 2010;31:29–34.

114. O'Keefe JH, Carter MD, Lavie CJ. Primary and secondary prevention of cardiovascular diseases: a practical evidence-based approach. Mayo Clin Proc 2009;84:741–57.

115. Esposito K, Giugliano F, Di Palo C, et al. Effect of lifestyle changes on erectile dysfunction in obese men. JAMA 2004;291(24):2978–84.

116. Giugliano D, Giugliano F, Esposito K. Sexual dysfunction and the Mediterranean diet. Public Health Nutr 2006;9:1118–20.

117. Critchley JA, Capewell S. Mortality risk reduction associated with smoking cessation in patients with coronary heart disease: a systematic review. JAMA 2003;290:86–97.

118. Plaskon LA, Penson DF, Vaughan TL, et al. Cigarette smoking and risk of prostate cancer in middle-aged men. Cancer Epidemiol Biomarkers Prev 2003;12:604–9.

119. Roberts WW, Platz EA, Walsh PC. Association of cigarette smoking with extraprostatic prostate cancer in young men. J Urol 2003;169:512–6.

120. Rodriguez C, Tatham LM, Thun MJ, et al. Smoking and fatal prostate cancer in a large cohort of adult men. Am J Epidemiol 1997;145:466–75.

121. Horasanli K, Boylu U, Kendirci M, et al. Do lifestyle changes work for improving erectile function? Asian J Androl 2008;10:28–35.

122. Mukamal KJ, Conigrave KM, Mittleman MA, et al. Roles of drinking pattern and type of alcohol consumed in coronary heart disease in men. N Engl J Med 2003;348:109–18.

123. Platz EA, Willet WC, Colditz GA, et al. Proportion of colon cancer risk that might be preventable in a cohort of middle-aged US men. Cancer Causes Control 2000;11:579–88.

124. Trichopoulou A, Costacou T, Bamia C, et al. Adherence to a Mediterranean diet and survival in a Greek population. N Engl J Med 2003;348:2599–608.

125. Mitrou PN, Kipnis V, Thiebaut AC, et al. Mediterranean dietary pattern and prediction of all-cause mortality in a U.S. population: results from the NIH-AARP Diet and Health Study. Arch Intern Med 2007;167:2461–8.

126. Yusuf S, Hawken S, Ounpuu S, et al. Effect of potentially modifiable risk factors associated with myocardial infarction in 52 countries (the INTERHEART study): case-control study. Lancet 2004; 364:937–52.

127. Joshi P, Islam S, Pais P, et al. Risk factors for early myocardial infarction in South Asians compared with individuals in other countries. JAMA 2007; 297:286–94.

128. Wilcox BJ, He Q, Chen R, et al. Midlife risk factors and healthy survival in men. JAMA 2006;296:2343–50.

129. Yates LB, Djousse L, Kurth T, et al. Exceptional longevity in men: modifiable factors associated with survival and function to age 90 years. Arch Intern Med 2008;168:284–90.

130. Terry DF, Pencina MJ, Vasan RS, et al. Cardiovascular risk factors predictive for survival and morbidity-free survival in the oldest-old Framingham Heart Study participants. J Am Geriatr Soc 2005;53:1944–50.

131. Rock CL. Multivitamin-multimineral supplements: who uses them? Am J Clin Nutr 2007;85(Suppl): 277S–9S.

132. Barqawi A, Gamito E, O'Donnell C, et al. Herbal and vitamin supplement use in a prostate cancer screening population. Urology 2004;63:288–92.

133. Kristal AR, Arnold KB, Schenk JM, et al. Dietary patterns, supplement use, and the risk of symptomatic benign prostatic hyperplasia: results from the Prostate Cancer Prevention Trial. Am J Epidemiol 2008;167:925–34.

134. Muntwyler J, Hennekens CH, Manson JE, et al. Vitamin supplement use in a low-risk population of US male physicians and subsequent cardiovascular mortality. Arch Intern Med 2002;162:1472–6.

135. Giovannucci E, Chan AT. Role of vitamin and mineral supplementation and aspirin use in cancer survivors. J Clin Oncol 2010;28:4081–5.

136. Lawson KA, Wright ME, Subar A, et al. Multivitamin use and risk of prostate cancer in the National Institutes of Health-AARP Diet and Health Study. J Natl Cancer Inst 2007;99:754–64.

137. Stevens VL, McCullough ML, Diver WR, et al. Use of multivitamins and prostate cancer mortality in a large cohort of US men. Cancer Causes Control 2005;16:643–50.

138. Neuhouser ML, Barnett MJ, Kristal AR, et al. Dietary supplement use and prostate cancer risk in the Carotene and Retinol Efficacy Trial. Cancer Epidemiol Biomarkers Prev 2009;18:2202–6.

139. Larsson SC, Akesson A, Bergkvist L, et al. Multivitamin use and breast cancer incidence in a prospective cohort of Swedish women. Am J Clin Nutr 2010;91:1268–72.

140. Berube S, Diorio C, Brisson J. Multivitamin-multimineral supplement use and mammographic breast density. Am J Clin Nutr 2008;87:1400–4.

141. Clarke R, Halsey J, Lewington S, et al. Effects of lowering homocysteine levels with B vitamins on cardiovascular disease, cancer, and cause-specific mortality. Arch Intern Med 2010;170:1622–31.

142. Collin SM, Metcalfe C, Refsum H, et al. Circulating folate, vitamin B12, homocysteine, vitamin B12 transport proteins, and risk of prostate cancer: a case-control study, systematic review, and meta-analysis. Cancer Epidemiol Biomarkers Prev 2010;19:1632–42.

143. Ng K, Meyerhardt JA, Chan JA, et al. Multivitamin use is not associated with cancer recurrence or survival in patients with stage III colon cancer: findings from CALGB 89803. J Clin Oncol 2010;28:4354–63.

144. Hercberg S, Galan P, Preziosi P, et al. The SU.VI.MAX study: a randomized, placebo-controlled trial of the health effects of antioxidant vitamins and minerals. Arch Intern Med 2004;164:2335–42.

145. Meyer F, Galan P, Douville P, et al. Antioxidant vitamin and mineral supplementation and prostate cancer prevention in the SU.VI.MAX trial. Int J Cancer 2005;116:182–6.

146. Christen WG, Gaziano JM, Hennekens CH. Design of Physicians' Health Study II-a randomized trial of beta-carotene, vitamins E and C, and multivitamins, in prevention of cancer, cardiovascular disease, and eye disease, and review of results of completed trials. Ann Epidemiol 2000;10:125–34.

147. Barnett CM, Nielson CM, Shannon J, et al. Serum 25-OH vitamin D levels and risk of developing prostate cancer in older men. Cancer Causes Control 2010;21:1297–303.

148. Michaelsson K, Baron JA, Snellman G, et al. Plasma vitamin D and mortality in older men: a community-based prospective cohort study. Am J Clin Nutr 2010;92:841–8.

149. Sanders KM, Stuart AL, Williamson EJ, et al. Annual high-dose oral vitamin D and falls and fractures in older women. JAMA 2010;303:1815–22.

150. Bischoff-Ferrari HA, Giovannucci E, Willett WC, et al. Estimation of optimal serum concentrations of 25-hydroxyvitamin D for multiple health outcomes. Am J Clin Nutr 2006;84:18–28.

151. Zerwekh JE. Blood biomarkers of vitamin D status. Am J Clin Nutr 2008;87(Suppl):1087S–91S.

152. Isenor JE, Ensom MH. Is there a role for therapeutic drug monitoring of vitamin D level as a surrogate marker for fracture risk. Pharmacotherapy 2010;30:254–64.

153. Moyad MA. Why a statin and/or another proven heart healthy agent should be utilized in the next major cancer chemoprevention trial: part I. Urol Oncol 2004;22:466–71.

154. Moyad MA. Why a statin and/or another proven heart healthy agent should be utilized in the next major cancer chemoprevention trial: part II. Urol Oncol 2004;22:472–7.

155. Moyad MA. Heart healthy equals prostate healthy equals statins: the next cancer chemoprevention trial. Part I. Curr Opin Urol 2005;15:1–6.

156. Moyad MA. Heart healthy equals prostate healthy equals statins: the next cancer chemoprevention trial. Part II. Curr Opin Urol 2005;15:7–12.

157. Ridker PM, Danielson E, Fonseca FA, et al. Rosuvastatin to prevent vascular events in men and women with elevated C-reactive protein. N Engl J Med 2008;359:2195–207.

158. Everett BM, Glynn RJ, MacFadyen JG, et al. Rosuvastatin in the prevention of stroke among men and women with elevated levels of C-reactive protein: Justification for the Use of Statins in Prevention: an Intervention Trial Evaluating Rosuvastatin (JUPITER). Circulation 2010;121:143–50.

159. Platz EA, Till C, Goodman PJ, et al. Men with low serum cholesterol have a lower risk of high-grade prostate cancer in the placebo arm of the Prostate Cancer Prevention Trial. Cancer Epidemiol Biomarkers Prev 2009;18:2807–13.

160. Murtola TJ, Visakorpi T, Lahtela J, et al. Statins and prostate cancer prevention: where we are now and future directions. Nat Clin Pract Urol 2008;5:376–87.

161. St Sauver JL, Jacobsen SJ, Jacobson DJ, et al. Statin use and decreased risk of benign prostatic enlargement and lower urinary tract symptoms. BJU Int 2011;107(3):443–50.

162. Dadkhah F, Safarinejad MR, Asgari MA, et al. Atorvastatin improves the response to sildenafil in hypercholesterolemic men with erectile dysfunction and not initially responsive to sildenafil. Int J Impot Res 2010;22:51–60.

163. Katz MS, Carroll PR, Cowan JE, et al. Association of statin and nonsteroidal anti-inflammatory drug use with prostate cancer outcomes: results from CaPSURE. BJU Int 2010;106:627–32.

Adult Male Health Risks Associated with Congenital Abnormalities

Terry W. Hensle, MD[a],*, Christopher M. Deibert, MD, MPH[b]

KEYWORDS

- Congenital abnormalities • Hypospadias • Cryptorchidism
- Posterior urethral valves • Transition

There are a number of congenital abnormalities of the genitourinary system that have a definable durable impact on the adult lives of those individuals affected. This occurs despite prompt and appropriate surgical and medical intervention during infancy and childhood. The list of these anomalies has decreased dramatically over the past 2 decades, mostly because of the impact of antenatal screening and termination. We look at 3 abnormalities that fall into this category, including relatively common problems of the newborn male, such as hypospadias and cryptorchidism, as well as a less common issue, posterior urethral valves. Although these disorders are most often treated early in childhood, the sequelae of each may last into adolescence and adulthood. The effects can be manifest in terms of sexual function, voiding function, fertility, and even psychosexual well-being. An understanding and awareness of the consequences of these 3 congenital abnormalities is paramount for the long-term care of the pediatric patient as he transitions to adolescence and adulthood. An understanding of the long-term risks associated with each of these congenital abnormalities can help in their long-term management, in affected patients.

HYPOSPADIAS

Hypospadias is one of the most common congenital abnormalities of the male infant and is caused by incomplete fusion of the urethral folds during embryogenic formation of the penile urethra. The failure of tubalization results in an abnormally positioned urethral opening on the ventral surface of the penis. The incidence of hypospadias has remained relatively constant over several decades despite some recent controversy concerning the affects of "endocrine disruptors," such as phthalates and bisphenol-A on the incidence of hypospadias.[1] The incidence of hypospadias, as obtained from the databases of the New York State Congenital Malformation registry, as well as the California Birth Defects Monitoring program, remains constant, at about 6 cases per 1000 live male births.[2,3] A demonstrable increase in hypospadias frequency has been seen in certain groups of individuals, and certain risk factors have been identified, such as increased maternal age,[4] fertility enhancement procedures (IVF),[5] and vegetarian diets (phytoestrogens).[6]

Endocrine disruptors have been manufactured for more than 50 years and are widely used in plastic bottles, vinyl floors, food wraps, cosmetics, medical products, and toys. Much of the concern focuses on the allegedly significant in utero exposure to these endocrine disruptors and subsequent effects on the developing fetus. There is no question that estrogenic compounds can be potent modulators of biochemical and physiologic function in high doses. The evidence, however,

The authors have nothing to disclose.

[a] Department of Urology, Columbia University College of Physicians and Surgeons, 699 Teaneck Road, Suite 103, Teaneck, NJ 07666, USA

[b] Department of Urology, Herbert Irving Cancer Center, 161 Fort Washington Avenue, HIP 11th Floor, New York, NY 10032, USA

* Corresponding author.

E-mail address: twhenslemd@aol.com

0094-0143/12/$ – see front matter © 2012 Elsevier Inc. All rights reserved.

that in utero or adult exposure to very low levels of environmental substances, such as phthalates and bisphenol-A, can produce any clinically detectable effects in the human is absent.[7]

The real question for clinicians is, does hypospadias in childhood affect sexual function, voiding function, and reproductive function in adulthood?

The Psychosocial Impact of Hypospadias in Adulthood

Publications looking at the psychosocial, sexual, and reproductive impact of hypospadias in patients operated on, using twenty-first century techniques, really do not exist. There are studies from the 1980s that suggest that, in adult men operated on for hypospadias during childhood, there was a less than satisfactory psychosocial adjustment as compared with age-matched controls. The patients with hypospadias were more timid and embarrassed and appeared to be more socially isolated as adults. They had lower self-esteem and decreased capacity for social and emotional relationships, as well as being less qualified for stressful occupations, when compared with a control population.

In 1989, Sandberg and colleagues[8] at Columbia University, in a study of 69 children with a history of hypospadias showed that these children had more behavioral problems and lower social skills than children in the general population. A number of older studies, including Sandberg and colleagues'[8] data, tend to support the fact that children of this era who had a history of multiple surgeries for hypospadias had less social competency than their peers. It was also found that children with hypospadias were less likely to verbalize their problems. In a more recent questionnaire-based review looking at the social and sexual life of adult patients operated on for hypospadias during childhood, the group with hypospadias and control group gave similar responses and did not differ in terms of success in sexual and social activities. Patients with hypospadias were more dissatisfied with the cosmetic results of their surgery than control patients, however, and they were more likely to have problems with urinary function.[9]

In another study of more than 11,000 men age 18 or older, there were 42 individuals with a history of hypospadias with a similar number of controls without hypospadias.[10] The hypospadias group was found to be significantly more inhibited in seeking sexual contacts and had a significantly lower number of patients who had already had full sexual intercourse by age 18. In addition, men with hypospadias were also significantly more likely than control patients to have a negative appraisal of their own genitalia. In terms of patient satisfaction with the cosmetic results of their surgery, the overwhelming majority of patients operated upon in childhood for hypospadias consider their penile appearance to be abnormal. Overall, patients with hypospadias seem to be somewhat less satisfied than their surgeons with the overall cosmetic appearance following hypospadias surgery.

All of these studies, however, included individuals who were operated on some years ago when hypospadias techniques were not as sophisticated as they are today and often involved operations over several years. The number of operations alone can have a significant impact on psychosocial development. The adult satisfaction rates will hopefully improve as the population that has undergone repairs with more modern techniques becomes adult and sexually active.

Micturition

Micturition after hypospadias repair has been reviewed in a number of studies,[10,11] and in general most report significantly more urinary issues than in controls. Most studies looking at voiding function in individuals operated on in childhood for hypospadias suggest that concerns generally include spraying of urination more than 50% of the time, as well as postvoid dribbling, and the feeling of incomplete emptying. In a few studies where a uroflow has been used to measure micturition, the Qmax was found to be abnormal in 13.5% of patients with hypospadias compared with 2.9% of controls.[11] In general, the more proximal the hypospadias, the more likely voiding issues were to occur. Recently, some concerns have been raised regarding long-term meatal issues in the TIP (Snodgrass) repair.

Ejaculation

In a number of studies from 1975 to 2000, there were difficulties with ejaculation reported in between 6% and 37% of individuals after hypospadias repair.[10,11] The problems included weak or dribbling ejaculation, retained ejaculate having to be expressed manually, and delayed ejaculation or anejaculation.[9] Once again, the more severe or proximal the original lesion, the more severe the ejaculatory issues.

Hypospadias in Adult Males

The surgical correction of hypospadias may at times be delayed for cultural, religious, or socioeconomic reasons. We have previously reported our experience with adult hypospadias repair, indicating the complexity of the surgical procedure and relatively poor outcome as compared with childhood hypospadias repair.[12] There is little information concerning impact on pychosocial development of these individuals or information about sexual function before or after correction. It has been reported that about 40% of adult patients with hypospadias have not attempted sexual intercourse before the operation.[13] Complications after childhood repairs, such as fistula and strictures, most often seen in the immediate postoperative period, can develop late and be seen in the adult. These complications are not simply missed problems in childhood but, de novo events in the adult. The correction of late complications is not straightforward, and clear disclosure of the complexity of repair must be given to the patient.

Reproduction

Hypospadias is frequently associated with other genitourinary abnormalities, the most common being undescended testis, which ranges between 17% and 30% of patients born with hypospadias.[14] The frequency of undescended testis varies with the severity of hypospadias and may be as high as 31% in severe forms of hypospadias. The frequency of undescended testis in the general population ranges between 3% and 5%[15] and is reported to be between 5% and 10% of individuals presenting with infertility.[16] Testicular atrophy is a known feature (complication) of surgery for undescended testis and testicular atrophy is obviously a risk factor for impaired infertility. Older literature suggests there may be abnormal levels of follicle-stimulating hormone in individuals with undescended testis and hypospadias; however, recent findings in 32 children with isolated hypospadias indicated that none of the patients presented with enzymatic abnormalities of testosterone biosynthesis or partial androgen insensitivity.[17]

What is clear from recent data is that most men with hypospadias alone have normal semen quality; however, semen quality is reduced for men with hypospadias plus other genital abnormalities, including undescended testis. Reproductive hormone levels indicate a subtle impairment of testicular function in men with hypospadias alone. It has been observed that there are fewer fathers among men with hypospadias versus controls. This may be because of several factors, including psychosocial factors, sexual dysfunction, reduced semen quality, or most likely a combination of all of these factors. In summary, there is no clear-cut association of hypospadias, undescended testis, and reduced fertility potential.

Summary

Studies outlining the long-term effects of hypospadias repair in childhood using modern twenty-first century techniques are scarce, but it seems clear that surgery in early childhood with better techniques will improve overall functional and cosmetic results long term. As far as micturition is concerned, adult patients with hypospadias have significantly more urinary symptoms when compared with adult controls and, in general, the more severe the primary lesion, the more severe are the micturition issues. In terms of cosmesis, the results of hypospadias repair done in childhood are generally good; however, there are a significant number of individuals who following their surgery will consider their penile appearance to be abnormal. In terms of sexuality, adult patients with hypospadias are generally reported to be less satisfied with sexual function when compared with controls. This lower satisfaction may be related to cosmesis, issues with body image, or low self-esteem. Erectile dysfunction is more prevalent in patients with hypospadias as compared with controls, and patients with severe hypospadias in particular report more ejaculatory problems than controls. In terms of relationships, adult patients born with severe hypospadias have fewer intimate relationships, lower self-esteem, negative genital appraisal, and inhibition in sexual contact as compared with controls.

UNDESCENDED TESTIS

Cryptorchidism is the most common congenital abnormality affecting the newborn male. The incidence is probably about 3% of all full-term male infants and as high as 30% in premature infant boys. Roughly 80% of cryptorchid testes will descend in the first 10 months of life and it is the remaining 20% that require our attention and monitoring. About two-thirds of the cases of undescended testis will be unilateral and about a third will involve both testes. In more than 90% of individuals, the undescended testis can be palpated either in the high portion of the scrotum or the inguinal canal, and the other 10% are nonpalpable.

The obvious ongoing concern for children born with undescended testes moving toward adolescence and adulthood is the impact of undescended testes on fertility potential and the development of testicular germ cell tumors. The temperature effects on the undescended testis affecting fertility potential have been well documented. The universal recommendation for early surgery is based on the studies showing degeneration of the germ cell population of the testis and reduced spermatogonia after the second year of life in the undescended testis. Despite this shift toward early surgery for undescended testis, there is no good data to judge whether fertility impairment has been prevented or improved by early orchidopexy. The fertility impairment in individuals born with a unilateral undescended testis is, if anything mild. In cases of bilateral cryptorchidism, however, there is reported to be a reduced fertility potential of more than 30% or 6 times that of the general population, even after treatment. In individuals with a small testis at orchidopexy, there is a clear association between the subnormal testicular volume and reduced fertility in adulthood.[18]

The other ongoing concern associated with cryptorchidism is the associated testicular cancer risk. What is unknown is whether the condition of maldescent predisposes to dysplasia of the testis in fetal life. To look at the question of cryptorchidism and testis cancer, Wood and Elder[19] have produced a thorough review of the subject in which they looked at a number of questions concerning testis cancer and cryptorchidism. Their data would suggest a significant increased relative risk of testis cancer in all individuals born with undescended testis. The relative risk is reduced markedly in patients undergoing prepubertal orchidopexy. They note a higher relative risk for patients with bilateral undescended testes and a higher relative risk for retained intra-abdominal testes versus retained inguinal testes. They also clearly demonstrate that the relative risk of the contralateral normally descended testis is no different than the general population. All of these findings are significant for clinicians following these children born with undescended testes into adulthood.

The question of whether testis location affects pathologic subtype of tumors when they occur is intriguing. The review by Wood and Elder[19] would suggest that about three-quarters of the tumors developing in uncorrected abdominal or inguinal testis are seminoma, whereas more than 60% of the tumors developing in testes that had been surgically lowered are diagnosed as nonseminomatous tumors. The associated question therefore would be, does orchidopexy decrease the risk of testis cancer in the previously undescended testis? The known literature would suggest that prepubertal orchidopexy (before age 10–12 years) does decrease the relative risk of testis cancer as compared with orchidopexy after the age of 12. What is not available are data to show whether early orchidopexy (before age 2), as done today, is going to impart greater protection from testis tumor than previous data would suggest. The

last question addressed in the review by Wood and Elder[19] is whether a testicular nubbin left after a perinatal torsion is at risk of malignant degeneration. Their data and data from the literature would suggest that only about 10% of these nubbins contain seminiferous tubules and very few have viable germ cells, therefore the risk of malignant degeneration is minimal, if present at all.

The take-home message for clinicians monitoring individuals who have been born with cryptorchidism would be to know the anatomic position of the cryptorchid testis before treatment and the age at which treatment was rendered. The potential for malignant degeneration in these individuals has to be discussed with the patient and the family going forward from childhood to the adult world.

Posterior Urethral Valves

One of the most devastating congenital anomalies in the male infant is posterior urethral valves (PUV), which cannot only affect long-term bladder function, but also renal function in a significant number of the individuals so effected. The incidence of PUV ranges from 1 in 4000 to 1 in 7500 live male births. The postnatal sequelae range from minor to life threatening. The impact of this anomaly can involve relatively simple problems with lower urinary tract function with incontinence to devastating issues with chronic renal insufficiency and end-stage renal disease (ESRD). Total bladder outlet bladder obstruction by PUV before 20 weeks of gestation has been shown to result in bilateral renal dysplasia and severe pulmonary hypoplasia, leading to death (Potter syndrome). Less than complete obstruction often leads to varying degrees of bladder dysfunction and/or renal damage. The incidence of newborns with PUV has decreased dramatically over 20 years, most probably because of antenatal screening and early termination. There has been a significant amount of interest generated over the past 3 decades in antenatal screening and intervention for PUV. The most common intervention to date has been the vesicoamniotic shunt. The long-term results are not convincing in terms of any real benefit being added by the use of antenatal shunting. Although there is some evidence that bladder function and perhaps renal function can be salvaged by early intervention and decompression, the pulmonary injury has not shown to be effected in a positive way. There are scattered reports of individual successes; however, long-term data to date are not terribly hopeful.[20]

There are few if any data to suggest that the initial approach to PUV makes any difference whatsoever in terms of long-term renal function and progression to ESRD. Most reports suggest that primary valve ablation and allowing the bladder to cycle is superior to primary supravesical diversion in terms of normalizing long-term bladder function. In addition, there are no data to suggest that the upper tract outcome is any different in children who have had prenatal intervention as compared with those who have had early postnatal intervention.[21]

Posterior Urethral Valves and End-Stage Renal Disease

Obstructive uropathy, which is caused by posturethral valves, continues to be a common cause of chronic renal insufficiency in children and adolescents. The rate of progression of renal insufficiency to ESRD in these children with PUV is probably somewhere between 13% and 20%.[22] The most important prognostic factor in these children going forward is their nadir serum creatinine. A serum creatinine of less than 0.8 mg/dL at 1 year of age is associated with essentially normal long-term real function, whereas a nadir creatinine of greater than 1.2 mg/dL after 12 months of age has a much more rapid acceleration to ESRD.[23] Findings would suggest that, in most boys, the die for ultimate renal function is cast at presentation. Those with good renal function will do well and those with poor renal function will not. The time frame for ESRD is largely dependent on the level of renal function to begin with. In most situations, the time to progression ranges between 11 and 15 years, which corresponds with pubertal development. The other important cofactors affecting the rate of progression to ESRD would include high-grade vesicoureteral reflux and persistent bladder dysfunction.

Posterior Urethral Valves and Bladder Dysfunction

Bladder dysfunction has an enormous impact not only on toilet training in children with PUV but also on progression to ESRD. Most clinicians agree that the long-term outcome in patients with PUV revolves around the management of their bladder dysfunction. It has been estimated that up to 75% of children born with PUV have underlying bladder dysfunction in spite of adequate valve fulguration early on.[22] The long-term use of clean intermittent catheterization, as well as the use of anticholinergics, can be extremely helpful in these patients, especially those with more chronic and slow renal deterioration caused by increased bladder pressure. In addition, Koff and colleagues[24] have shown that overnight bladder drainage will further decrease bladder dysfunction, lower intravesical pressure, and delay renal insufficiency.

The bladder dysfunction seen in patients with PUV in association with ongoing renal deterioration has been labeled the "valve bladder syndrome." This is characterized by myogenic failure of the bladder with poor compliance and detrusor hyperactivity. The renal failure seen in conjunction with the valve/bladder syndrome is characterized by a lack of concentrating ability, leading to increased urine production. This association was noted first by Mitchell in 1982.[25] It is exceedingly important that clinicians following patients with PUV understand that the valve bladder is not stable. It has been noted for a long time that valve bladders that are hypocompliant in infancy and early childhood can decompensate rather rapidly in adolescent years. This is extremely important in following these patients through adolescence. The typical urodynamic patterns seen in adolescent patients with valve/bladders include hyperreflexia, hypertonia, and myogenic failure.

The other significant change that has taken place in the management of these individuals born with PUV is the sharp reduction in the use of augmentation cystoplasty. In our database, which encompasses 33 years of data collection, there are 157 augmentation cystoplasties and 91 continent diversions. Of that number, 24 of the augmentation cystoplasties were in patients with PUV, including 19 gastric cystoplasties and 6 ureterocystoplasties; however, since 2000, there have been only 3 augmentation cystoplasties done in patients with PUV at our institution, and each of the 3 were patients referred long into the course of their treatment (Hensle, unpublished data, 2001). This decrease in the use of augmentation cystoplasty reflects the better management of the high-pressure noncompliant bladder with anticholinergics, clean intermittent catheterization, and overnight drainage.[26]

In patients with ESRD secondary to posterior urethral valves, renal transplantation into valve/bladders has shown to be safe in a number of recent studies.[27] These studies have concluded that a history of PUV does not portend a worse prognosis for renal graft survival compared with individuals transplanted for nonvalve issues. In patients with a valve bladder undergoing transplantation, the treatment plan has to be individualized to prevent lower tract deterioration. This often includes intermittent catheterization, anticholinergics, and overnight drainage. This allowed safe and effective renal transplantation in those individuals requiring it.[28,29]

The single most important feature in dealing with these children as they move to adolescence and adulthood is to customize the urologic management of their bladder to decrease the risk of ongoing renal insufficiency and make success of renal transplantation optimal. This often requires close monitoring of these individuals with frequent video urodynamic evaluations and attention to detail in terms of the individual's commitment to clean-intermittent catheterization and, if appropriate, nocturnal urinary drainage. What is of critical importance to the clinical urologist following these youngsters as they move from childhood to adolescence to adulthood with a hostile bladder is to be sure that the bladder management in terms of filling, emptying, and pressure management is under good control to protect what is either left of native renal function or to protect the native or transplanted kidney.

REFERENCES

1. Wang M, Baskin L. Endocrine disrupters, genital development, and hypospadias. J Androl 2008; 29(5):499–505.
2. Choi J, Cooper KL, Hensle TW, et al. Incidents and surgical repair rates of hypospadias in New York State. Urology 2001;57:151–3.
3. Fisch H, Lambert SM, Hensle TW, et al. Hypospadias rates in New York State are not increasing. J Urol 2009;181:2291–4.
4. Fisch H, Golden RJ, Libersen GL, et al. Maternal age as a risk factor for hypospadias. J Urol 2001;165:934.
5. Silver R, Rodriguez R, Chang TSK, et al. In vitro fertilization is associated with an increased risk of hypospadias. J Urol 1999;161:1954.
6. North K, Golding J. A maternal estrogen diet in pregnancy is associated with hypospadias. The ALSPAC study team. Avon longitudinal study of pregnancy in childhood. BJU Int 2000;85:107.
7. Fisch H, Hyun G, Hensle TW. Rising hypospadias rates: disproving a myth. J Pediatr Urol 2010;6(1): 37–9.
8. Sandberg DE, Meyer-Bahlbeurg HF, Aranoff GS, et al. Boys with hypospadias: a survey of behavioral difficulties. J Pediatr Psychol 1989;14(4):491–514.
9. Rynja SP, DeJong TPV, Bosch JL, et al. Functional, cosmetic and psychological results in adult men who underwent hypospadias correction in childhood. J Pediatr Urol 2011;7(5):504–15.
10. Mondaninin N, Ponchietti R, Bonafem M, et al. Hypospadias: incidence and effects on psychosocial development as evaluated with the Minnesota Multiphasic Personality Inventory Test in a sample of 11,649 young Italian men. Urol Int 2002;68(2):81–5.
11. Mieusset R, Soulie M. Hypospadias: psychological, sexual and reproductive consequences in adult life. J Androl 2005;26(2):163–8.
12. Hensle TW, Tennenbaum SY, Reiley EA, et al. Hypospadias repair in adults: adventures and misadventures. J Urol 2001;165:77–9.
13. Moudouni S, Tanzi K, Nouri M, et al. Hypospadias in the adult. Prog Urol 2001;11:667–9.
14. Khun FJ, Hardy BE, Churchill BM. Urologic abnormalities associated with hypospadias. Urol Clin North Am 1981;8:565–71.
15. Thonnean PF, Gandia P, Mieusset R. Cryptorchidism: incidents, risk factors and potential role of environment: an update. J Androl 2003;24:155–62.
16. Carizza C, Anitba A, Palazzi J, et al. Testicular maldescent and infertility. Andrologia 1990;22:285–8.
17. Feyaerts A, Forest M, Morel Y, et al. Endocrine screening in 32 consecutive patients with hypospadias. J Urol 2002;168:720–5.
18. Lee P, Coughlin M, Bellinger M. No relationship with testicular size at orchiopexy with fertility in men who previously had unilateral cryptorchidism. J Urol 2001;166:236–9.
19. Wood H, Elder JS. Cryptorchidism and testicular cancer: separating fact from fiction. J Urol 2009; 181:452–61.
20. Aoba T, Kitagawa H, Pringle K, et al. Can a pressure limited vesicoamniotic shunt tube preserve normal bladder function? J Pediatr Surg 2008;43:2250–5.
21. DeFoor W, Curtis C, Jackson E, et al. Risk factors for end stage renal disease in children with posterior urethral valves. J Urol 2008;180:1705–8.
22. Ansari MS, Gulia A, Srivastava A, et al. Risk factors for progression to end stage renal disease in children with posterior urethral valves. J Pediatr Urol 2010;6:261–4.
23. Podesta M, Ruarte AC, Gargiulo R, et al. Bladder function associated with posterior urethral valves after primary valve ablation or proximal urinary diversion in children and adolescents. J Urol 2002;168: 1830–3.
24. Koff S, Mutabagani KH, Jayanthi VR. The valve bladder syndrome: pathophysiology and treatment with nocturnal bladder emptying. J Urol 2002;167:291–7.
25. Mitchell ME. Persistent urethral dilation following valve resection. Dialogues in Ped Urol 1982;5:8.
26. Lendvay TS, Cowan CA, Mitchell ME, et al. Augmentation cystoplasty rates in children's hospitals in the United States: a Pediatric Health Information System Database Study. J Urol 2006;176:1716–20.
27. Fine M, Smith KM, Shrivastava D, et al. Posterior urethral valve treatments and outcomes in children receiving kidney transplants. J Urol 2011;185: 2507–11.
28. Mendizabal S, Estornell F, Zamora I, et al. Renal transplantation in children with severe bladder dysfunction. J Urol 2005;173:226–9.
29. Solomon L, Fontaine E, Gagnoloux M, et al. Posterior urethral valves: long-term renal function consequences after transplantation. J Urol 1997;157:992–5.

Index

Note: Page numbers of article titles are in **boldface** type.

0094-0143/12/$ – see front matter © 2012 Elsevier Inc. All rights reserved.

urologic.theclinics.com

Moving?

Make sure your subscription moves with you!

To notify us of your new address, find your **Clinics Account Number** (located on your mailing label above your name), and contact customer service at:

Email: journalscustomerservice-usa@elsevier.com

800-654-2452 (subscribers in the U.S. & Canada)
314-447-8871 (subscribers outside of the U.S. & Canada)

Fax number: 314-447-8029

Elsevier Health Sciences Division
Subscription Customer Service
3251 Riverport Lane
Maryland Heights, MO 63043

*To ensure uninterrupted delivery of your subscription, please notify us at least 4 weeks in advance of move.

Printed and bound by CPI Group (UK) Ltd, Croydon, CR0 4YY

03/10/2024

01040350-0020